HYSTERECTOMY

Sandra Coney   Lyn Potter

Illustrations by Sharon Alston

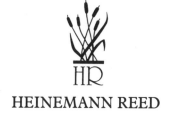

HEINEMANN REED

Published by Heinemann Reed, a division of Octopus Publishing Group (NZ) Ltd,
39 Rawene Road, Birkenhead, Auckland. Associated companies, branches and
representatives throughout the world.

ISBN 0 7900 0089 X
© 1990, Sandra Coney and Lyn Potter
First published May 1990
Reprinted November 1990

Designed by Kate Greenaway
Typeset by Rennies Illustrations Ltd
Printed in Singapore

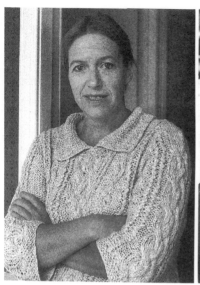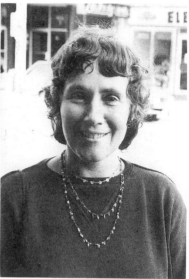

Sandra Coney (left) has worked on women's issues since the early 1970s, specialising in health. In 1971 she was one of a women's liberation group which ran a telephone contraceptive counselling service, and in 1974 she began working as a counsellor at the first abortion clinic in New Zealand. She has a particular interest in safe contraception, and in 1984, together with Phillida Bunkle, founded Fertility Action, a women's health consumer advocacy group. She is also an active member of the Auckland Women's Health Council, a powerful consumer lobby.

In 1987 Sandra Coney and Phillida Bunkle wrote the article which precipitated the Cervical Cancer Inquiry, about which Coney has written the award-winning book, *The Unfortunate Experiment*. Coney works as a freelance journalist, and has won a number of journalism awards.

Born in Auckland in 1944, Coney has two adult sons, likes gardening, eating and physical exercise. *(Photograph by Gil Hanly.)*

Lyn Potter (right) has been involved in health politics for the last

10 years. She is a member of the Auckland Women's Health Council. She is also on the Ministerial Committee on Women's Health and has been a member of the Auckland Area Health Board.

Because Lyn has a positive attitude to life, she was surprised that the hysterectomy that she had 10 years ago was such a bad experience. After having the operation she organised a Hysterectomy Support Group, and helped prepare a pamphlet on the subject for National Women's Hospital. She is grateful that good health since then has allowed her to explore new opportunities, and to enjoy family and friends.

Lyn lives in Auckland with her husband and three children.

CONTENTS

CONTENTS

ACKNOWLEDGEMENTS

We would like to thank the *New Zealand Woman's Weekly*, especially the then news editor, Pauline Ray, for publishing our questionnaire, and all the women who replied to it.

We owe a special and very considerable debt of gratitude to Lynne Giddings and Pamela Wood, nursing specialists, and David A. Weir, a computer specialist. When we received nearly 1 000 responses to our questionnaire we were thrilled, but we were also considerably daunted because analysing it would be a major task. Our many efforts to gain assistance from New Zealand universities and the Department of Health were fruitless. Just when we despaired of ever getting the analysis done, Lynne, Pamela and David offered to do the work, which they accomplished speedily and very ably. In addition, Lynne helped with other aspects of writing the book since she shared with us a commitment to this project. We are especially grateful to her.

Jill Bonham, staff nurse at National Women's Hospital, helped with the section on hospital procedures. Professor John Hutton, head of the Department of Obstetrics and Gynaecology at Wellington Women's Hospital, assisted with information and provided the photographs used in this book. We would also like to thank the women who allowed photographs to be taken. We were helped by Dr Paul Hutchison, an Auckland gynaecologist, who commented on the manuscript, and Professor Colin Mantell, head of the Department of Obstetrics and Gynaecology at Auckland Medical School. Valuable advice was given by Dr Klim McPherson of the Department of Community Medicine and General Practice at University of Oxford, who has done a good deal of epidemiological research on hysterectomy. He read parts of the manuscript. Dr Wendy Savage of London Hospital

Medical College and Diony Young of the International Childbirth Education Association also helped. Floris de Groot of the Auburn Centre provided information on depression and grief.

The preparation and publication of this survey and book were assisted by funds granted by the Roy McKenzie Foundation. However, the Roy McKenzie Foundation is not the author, publisher or proprietor of this publication and is not to be understood necessarily as approving by virtue of its grant any of the statements made or views expressed therein.

Finally, we would like to thank our editors, Linda Cassells and Chris Price, for their support and patience!

1

HOW THIS BOOK GOT WRITTEN

When one of us, Lyn, had a hysterectomy eight years ago, she badly needed but failed to find the right kind of information. She wanted to know more about what the surgery involved and under what circumstances it was really necessary. She would also have liked to have known about different women's experiences and how hysterectomy had affected them.

This is the kind of information we have tried to provide in this book. It is written for women who are considering a hysterectomy and also for women who have had one and who still have unanswered questions. We hope that doctors will read this book so that they have more information to pass on to their patients.

We met when Sandra was editing the feminist magazine *Broadsheet* and Lyn wrote an article about her hysterectomy experience and efforts to work with staff of Auckland's National Women's Hospital to produce a patient information leaflet on hysterectomy. Sandra has worked on women's health issues since the early seventies and Lyn worked as a telephone counsellor for hysterectomy patients.

In April 1987 the *New Zealand Woman's Weekly* published an article about our plan to write a book on hysterectomy. With it was published a questionnaire. Nine hundred and eighty-seven women completed and returned the questionnaire, making this survey very large indeed. The women's ages ranged from 35 to 84 years at the time of completing the questionnaire. The majority of the women (68 percent) were aged 30-44 years at the time of the operation, with the largest group (26 percent) aged 35-39 years.

Only two women were over 65, while 9 percent were under 30. The major reasons the younger women had hysterectomies did not differ markedly from those of the older women; they were heavy bleeding, fibroids and prolapse. But hysterectomy following problems after contraception use was more frequent among younger women. There were three women who were only 19 at the time of the operation. The reasons they gave were infection, endometriosis, and an emergency at the time of Caesarian section.

This survey gave us an amazing glimpse into the lives and feelings of New Zealand women. Many respondents supplied their names and addresses to show their good faith, although we had not requested this. A large number also wrote additional material and we have drawn from these experiences extensively. We are very grateful to all the women who helped us in this way. Their contribution has helped make this book different from overseas handbooks on hysterectomy. The themes that emerged from what women told us shaped the book and the issues we have tried to cover.

The questionnaire drew very few responses from Maori and Pacific Island women, despite the fact that 31 percent of Maori women and 27 percent of Pacific Island women read the *New Zealand Woman's Weekly*. (The figure for Pakeha women is 32.5 percent.) This may reflect the fact that fewer of these women have hysterectomies, but the more likely reason is that Maori and Pacific Island women do not feel comfortable about sharing personal information in this way.

Minority women such as lesbians and disabled women did not identify themselves, with two exceptions. We hope these women will still find our book useful, but it is unfortunate that we were unable to include their particular perspectives.

New Zealand has one of the highest hysterectomy rates in the world. One in four New Zealand women will have a hysterectomy before the age of 50. This is an alarming statistic. Our survey showed it was not uncommon for women to go ahead with surgery without fully understanding why hysterectomy had been suggested in the first place. It would also appear that many doctors glossed over any potential problems and virtually guaranteed them an excellent outcome. The foundation of this book is the need for 'informed consent', that is, the need for women to make their decisions knowing the possible risks and benefits.

We feel that with better information, hysterectomy rates will come down. Some women will opt for different forms of treatment and others may decide that their symptoms are preferable to the cure. This is not to say that we are *against* hysterectomy. But we are against unnecessary hysterectomy and we are certainly *for* fully informed choices.

For some women hysterectomy will be their preferred option. It can make a dramatic improvement in a woman's quality of life — many of the letters we received were testimony to this — but this does need to be balanced against the possibility of some unpleasant after-effects and the possibility that not all problems will be solved by the operation.

There is another reason why hysterectomy patients should have full information. Recent research has shown that patients who are well informed are less likely to become depressed and will have a better sexual adjustment. A programme at the Hasharon Hospital in Israel was reported at the International Congress on Menopause held in Belgium in 1981. In this hospital, women were given a pamphlet about how the surgery would be done and about hospital procedures. In addition they and their partners were invited to attend a group session at which the techniques used in vaginal and abdominal operations were explained. Information about the menstrual cycle and menopause was given and the relationship between hysterectomy and sexuality was emphasised. The evaluation showed a significantly better adjustment to hysterectomy for patients who attended these sessions. They were also very popular and so were continued by the hospital on a regular basis.

New Zealand hospitals hold antenatal classes for pregnant women and some provide information evenings for infertile women, but very little is done for hysterectomy patients, despite the fact that this is common and major surgery. In addition, the written material that we have surveyed was generally sketchy and patronising in tone. We hope this book will help women to be more knowledgeable and assertive. As Lyn says, 'From my experience, it doesn't pay to be a mouse.'

Hysterectomy is a major event in women's lives. This was illustrated by the fact that some women wrote to us about hysterectomies that had taken place 40 or 50 years ago. It seems extraordinary that women have known so little about an operation that so many have had. With the publication of this book, we hope this will come to an end.

2

THE UTERUS, ITS NEIGHBOURS, AND HOW THEY WORK

The uterus, or womb as it is commonly called, is a unique organ. It is deep inside a woman's body, yet it can be seen and felt from the 'outside' at the top of the vagina. It is soft and vulnerable to damage and infection, yet tough enough to stretch to many times its normal size during pregnancy and withstand the violent contractions of childbirth. It also changes dramatically during the course of a woman's life. When a female child is born, the uterus is tiny, but during puberty it will enlarge and begin to bleed. It can help to transform a tiny zygote formed from a microscopic ovum and sperm into a healthy living child, expelled fully functioning into the world. With age it will shrink to its prepubescent size.

Although doctors, scientists and philosophers have written about the uterus for thousands of years, there are still mysteries about the way the uterus functions. Menstruation and ovulation and the interrelationships between the uterus, ovaries and other body organs are still imperfectly understood.

The versatile womb

The uterus lies inside the girdle of pelvic bones, which also hold the bladder and rectum. It sits closely between these two organs

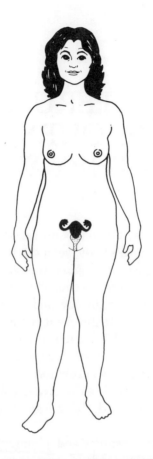

Position and size of the uterus and ovaries in a woman's body.

so that a problem with the uterus may manifest itself in problems with urination or bowel motions. Above it lie the coils of the bowel, and below it the vagina. It is frequently compared in shape to a pear or a light bulb and in an adult non-pregnant woman is about as big as these objects.

There is a cavity inside the uterus, which in a non-pregnant woman is a potential space rather than an actual one, a bit like the space in an empty hot-water bottle. In a non-pregnant woman this cavity is tiny — not much bigger than a thumb-nail.

The outside of the uterus is covered in a smooth skin-like layer called peritoneum. Almost 90 percent of the uterus is made up of thick muscled walls. These strong muscles, unlike muscles in the arms or legs, cannot be controlled at will. They function in response to chemical messages from hormones and the nervous system. The function of the muscles is to expel a child or menstrual blood. The muscle contractions of the uterus are very strong — the pressure reached is only one-third less than the pressure the heart uses to pump blood right around the body.

Women may be conscious of the uterus at other times. Some women experience pleasurable uterine contractions during orgasm or when their nipples are fondled during love-making. One of the respondents to our questionnaire said that after surgery there was 'totally no reaction from breast stimulation which was once a very pleasurable part of my love life'. A woman may feel a reaction in her uterus when suckling her baby and breastfeeding helps the uterus to contract to its non-pregnant size. These experiences underline the complex way in which women's bodies function, a complexity sometimes denied by medical attitudes to the reproductive organs.

Getting to know the womb

The fatter part of the uterus is called the fundus (base), even though it lies at the top in a woman's body. The smaller end, poking down into the vagina, is called the cervix (neck) and the passage through the cervix into the interior of the uterus is the cervical canal. The opening of the cervical canal into the vagina is called the os (mouth). The cervix can be felt at the end of the vagina as a smooth hard knob, a bit like the end of your nose. Women who use a diaphragm or cervical cap as contraception need to be able to feel their cervices. Using a speculum, an

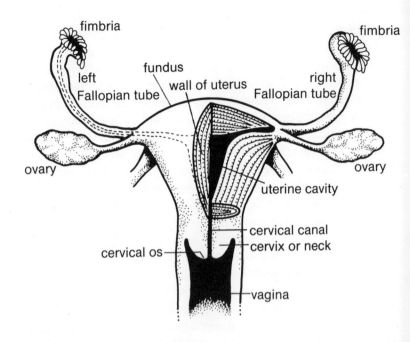

Female reproductive organs.

instrument shaped rather like a duck's bill, which holds the vaginal walls open, it is possible to see one's own cervix. Well women's centres sometimes teach this technique, which enables women to see if their cervices are healthy, and to detect pregnancy, when the cervix usually becomes blue in colour.

The muscle of the uterus is arranged in two patterns: muscles that run from the cervix over the fundus and back to the cervix again, which squeeze out the contents of the uterus, whether a baby or blood, and a criss-cross network of smaller muscles that shut off small blood vessels and therefore control bleeding at the end of menstruation or in childbirth.

The uterus is attached to the pelvis by ligaments, which are partly elastic tissue and partly muscle. They provide support, but allow for the uterus to move or grow within the pelvis. If these ligaments stretch through wear and tear, usually related to childbirth, the uterus will fall down. This is covered fully in chapter 4.

Variety in uteri

In about 80 percent of women the uterus tips forward over the bladder, and this is called anteverted. In the other 20 percent of women the uterus tips back towards the bowel. Women with this sort of uterus, called retroverted, sometimes become constipated because of pressure on the bowel or have backache.

As recently as 20 years ago, some women were told their retroverted uteri were abnormal and that they might have trouble conceiving. Operations were even performed to turn the uterus forwards. In fact a retroverted uterus is perfectly normal and rarely makes a difference to a woman's fertility. In some women the uterus will change position, being sometimes anteverted and sometimes retroverted. This is also perfectly normal.

The uterus normally changes position according to what the woman is doing. When her bowel or bladder is full the uterus will be pushed out of the way. When she lies down the uterus will settle back towards the spine and when she stands it will drop slightly. During sexual excitement the ligaments will pull the uterus upwards to make more room for the penis. Nevertheless, some women will feel the penis push the cervix during intercourse and if the uterus is pushed into an uncomfortable position there can be a sharp pain.

Occasionally, a woman has an unusual sort of uterus. She may have two cavities inside the uterus, even two cervical canals and two os. These have different medical names, but the most common is a bicornate uterus. In rare cases, a woman may have two uteri and two vaginas. This is not necessarily all bad: one woman told her doctor sexual intercourse felt different according to which vagina her husband put his penis in, and she could choose according to her mood!

Some uterine abnormalities can make it difficult for a woman to use an IUD, become pregnant or carry a pregnancy to term. One type, called a T-shaped uterus, has been found in the daughters of mothers who took a drug called DES during pregnancy.

The monthly cycle

The uterine cavity is lined with a mucous membrane called endometrium, which thickens and is shed each month as a menstrual period, unless pregnancy has occurred. Oestrogen released from the ovaries stimulates the endometrium so that new cells grow and develop. At this stage of the menstrual cycle the term proliferative endometrium is used to describe this normal thickening. When the oestrogen level drops, the endometrium dies and comes away as a period.

The cessation of menstrual bleeding depends on three factors: the closing of the small uterine muscles, which is prompted by hormone production; blood clotting; and the beginning of growth of a new endometrium. Because this bleeding is so complex, less is known about it than bleeding in other parts of the body. This complexity also means there is more to go wrong. If any of the systems are faulty, there can be excess bleeding. There is no point in treating excess bleeding with hormones if the cause is not hormonal.

There is a rich supply of nerves to the uterus and how these work is not fully understood. Messages carried from the brain to nerves connected to the cervix, blood vessels and muscle cells can affect the amount of blood flowing to the uterus and the actions of muscles. It has been suggested that the cutting of the nerves between the uterus and Fallopian tubes during therapeutic sterilisation may be responsible for the heavier menstrual bleeding some women experience after tubal ligation.

Tubes and ovaries

The Fallopian tubes are hollow tubes as big as drinking straws, and they link the uterus to the ovaries. One end of each is attached to the uterus on either side of the fundus while the other end is free, flaring outwards. Finger-like projections at this end, called fimbria, actually suck an ovum from the ovary and into the tube. The interior of the tube is narrow and lined with microscopic hairs called cilia, which by beating propel the ovum along the tube towards the uterus. If fertilisation occurs, it happens in the tube, when the ovum meets sperm that have swum up from the uterus. The fertilised egg slowly moves down the tube and embeds in the lining of the uterus. The delicate cilia are easily damaged by infection; tubal blockage is a common cause of infertility in women.

At the end of the two Fallopian tubes and attached to the uterus by ligaments are the ovaries. They are greyish-white and about the size of a prune. The ovaries have two functions. They store the ova and release one each month, and they produce the hormones oestrogen and progesterone, which control the menstrual cycle, promote female sexual characteristics such as breasts and rounded hips, and effect changes in the vagina, clitoris and labia during sexual excitement. Oestrogen production from the ovaries slowly decreases over our lives, reaching a low point at menopause that will continue till we are about 70. This loss of oestrogen is thought to be responsible for the loss of bone density in post-menopausal women called osteoporosis, sometimes leading to debilitating or even fatal fractures. Oestrogen loss can also cause thinning of the vaginal walls, loss of lubrication during sex, hot flushes and thinning of the skin.

The loss of one ovary, or even all of one and part of the other, does not mean that all oestrogen production will cease. Even part of one ovary can sometimes produce enough oestrogen to prevent the symptoms of oestrogen loss. Small amounts of oestrogen are also produced in body fat, which is one reason why women who are fat rarely develop osteoporosis. If both ovaries are removed in pre-menopausal women, oestrogen replacement therapy is usually suggested.

The change of life

As we reach menopause, which usually occurs in the mid- to late forties or early fifties, our hormones are often unevenly produced, resulting in hormonal disturbances such as hot flushes and changes in our periods. Some women have heavy bleeding and some women have light periods; for others the flow will vary from period to period. In addition, the periods may become irregular, they may be skipped or the time between them become erratic. Women should be aware of the difference between normal menopausal bleeding and abnormal bleeding. Flooding, bleeding between periods, very frequent periods or any bleeding after periods have stopped should be reported to a doctor, because they could be symptoms of disease.

Menopause is said to have occurred when a woman has had no menstrual bleeding for two years. Until this is achieved, she should take contraceptive precautions.

3

HYSTERECTOMY IN NEW ZEALAND

Around 7 000 hysterectomies are performed in this country every year, making hysterectomy the most common major operation for women. This was revealed in the *New Zealand Medical Journal* in June 1987 by researcher Mary Macintosh. She estimated that New Zealand women had an almost 40 percent chance of having a hysterectomy before the age of 85, and a 25 percent chance of having one before the age of 50. The New Zealand rate of 4.1 hysterectomies per 1 000 women in the population in 1984 was the second highest in the world, exceeded only by North America (5.6 in 1980) and far higher than England and Wales (2.4) Scotland (1.8) and somewhat higher than Australia (3.8).

These rates are averaged over all females, from babies upwards. Closer attention to age groups in figures provided by the National Health Statistics Centre shows that the highest rates are in the 35–50 year age groups, although the rate is also surprisingly high for women in their early thirties.

A 1988 study of contraceptive use among New Zealand women provided further confirmation of the country's high hysterectomy rate. Charlotte Paul found that 16 percent of women aged 35–44 had had a hysterectomy, as had 21 percent of women aged 45–54. She commented that the rate for women in their forties was exactly the same as that shown for US women.

While the rate in North America is steadily coming down (6.7 in 1975, 5.5 in 1985), the rate in New Zealand has stayed the same since the late seventies. It shows no signs of decreasing. In many parts of the world, for example North America, Britain, Australia and the Netherlands there is concern on the part of some doctors and women's groups at the high rates for this operation.

Macintosh found that (as in most countries) hysterectomy rates varied within New Zealand. South Canterbury (7.1) and Canterbury (6.3) had the highest rates. Auckland, Wellington, Waikato and Nelson were all similar at over 4 per 1 000 women.

Why so high?

There is no way of explaining New Zealand's higher hysterectomy rate or these regional differences without further study, and hysterectomy is not an area that has attracted much attention from New Zealand researchers, perhaps because it is not one of medicine's 'glamour' areas. It is possible but very unlikely that there is something different about New Zealand women. It has been suggested that the New Zealand diet, with the high consumption of red meats, may have something to do with the prevalence of bleeding problems as women get older. This is pure speculation and, of course, does not explain why women in one part of New Zealand are more likely than their sisters in other parts of the country to have a hysterectomy.

Macintosh points out that hysterectomy is 'discretionary surgery'. This means that doctors can choose to recommend it, so our higher hysterectomy rate probably reflects 'greater acceptance of hysterectomy for minor indications'. In 1984, 42 percent of hysterectomies were performed privately; in areas where there were no private hysterectomies the rate was half the national rate.

When feminists began working on women's health issues in the 1970s, they were critical of the increasing hysterectomy rate. They argued that some doctors operated for profit rather than as a result of real health indicators. In the USA, they quoted studies that showed that between 33 percent and 50 percent of hysterectomies were unnecessary. They talked about the 'hysterectomy industry' and called hysterectomy 'hip pocket surgery'.

In New Zealand, although the profit motive could account for some privately performed hysterectomies (hysterectomy is very expensive and therefore lucrative surgery), our rates are also high in public hospitals. Vicki Hufnagel, an American gynaecologist who wrote a book called *No More Hysterectomies*, argues that obstetrics and gynaecology as a branch of medicine includes few areas of major, lucrative surgery. Hysterectomy, she maintains, keeps doctors in work, whether they work publicly or privately. The Australian gynaecologist Dr Lorraine Dennerstein, who has written books on gynaecology and hysterectomy, says that 'hysterectomy is one of the few major operations done by the gynaecologist and pride, technical practice and financial incentive may generate a bias towards this'.

Medical professionals tend to trivialise the serious nature of the surgery and the loss of the organs involved. Women have succumbed to propaganda that hysterectomy is simple, even 'natural', a stage we go through after our families are completed.

Doctors who do and doctors who don't

Canadian research by Naralou Roos has shown that there are doctors who can be described as 'hysterectomy prone', and in Australia Opit and Gadiel found that 25 percent of doctors in New South Wales performed nearly 70 percent of the hysterectomies.

There is other research which shows that simply visiting a doctor increases a woman's chance of having surgery. Sonja McKinlay of the New England Research Institute in Massachusetts has been conducting a large study of mid-life women. The biggest predictor of a woman getting a hysterectomy, she says, is prior use of the health care system. Visiting the doctor increases the likelihood of hysterectomy. She found that women who had had hysterectomies were also twice as likely to have had breast surgery.

On the other hand, there are doctors who are opposed to hysterectomy, or very cautious about it. Some believe that women should put up with their problems and think that they complain too much. The attitude of individual doctors will be a key factor in whether they suggest hysterectomy for a given complaint.

One woman told us of her doctor's lack of interest in her complaints. She was first referred to a specialist for heavy periods when she was 15, but didn't actually have an internal examination until she was 30. She was simply given hormones by all the doctors she saw. When she was in her thirties she was bleeding seven days every fortnight and had fibroids diagnosed (probably encouraged by the oestrogen in the hormone therapy). She wrote: 'It does little for a woman's confidence (I am a professional woman dealing with the public) to be often bathed in blood and to be light-headed and shivery. When one goes through 40–50 super-plus tampons and the same number of maternity pads, it does little for one's equilibrium to have it suggested, yet again, that one should accept it as part of being a woman!'

Another wrote that she had had to have blood transfusions because of her blood loss during menstruation. When she told the hospital specialist that her own GP thought she needed a hysterectomy, he replied: 'You've had two children, what do you expect?' He prescribed more hormones, but would not recommend a hysterectomy. Finally she had the operation done privately.

There are some doctors who regard removal of the uterus as terrible. One woman told of a doctor being called in to look at her post-operative infection. ' "Well, you women who will go ahead and have destructive surgery . . ." he said to me. I found out his attitude was that women were on earth solely for reproductive purposes and therefore the womb is sacred!'

There has been virtually no research on doctors' attitudes to hysterectomy. One Swiss study of hysterectomy did ask questions to assess the effect of the sex of the gynaecologist on hysterectomy rates. It found that female gynaecologists performed half as many hysterectomies as their male colleagues in the same kind of medical practice. They speculated that women doctors might identify more easily with some women's negative view that hysterectomy signalled 'loss of womanhood and of attractiveness' and therefore might recommend it less often.

The 'worthless' womb

During the 1970s it became quite common for doctors in many countries to argue that the uterus was redundant after childbearing was completed. The uterus was seen simply as a receptacle for a baby. The part it played in sexual response, the desire of some women to continue menstruating, and the links between self-esteem and intact reproductive organs were all dismissed. Women who expressed these views might even be seen as irrational and unduly fearful. The uterus was an expendable organ, like an appendix or tonsil. It was depicted as a potential site for disease and thus better removed. A 'birthday hysterectomy' became almost routine for women turning 40. Experience in New Zealand and overseas showed that many of the uteruses removed turned out to be quite healthy with no abnormalities present.

The most extreme statement of the redundant uterus view, made by a Connecticut gynaecologist, has become quite infamous. Dr R. C. Wright said the uterus was 'a useless, bleeding, symptom-producing, potentially cancer-bearing organ and therefore should be removed'. He argued for universal removal of this 'lethal organ'.

New Zealand has not been immune to such trivialising attitudes. One woman told us her doctor said that in a hysterectomy, 'we remove the music box, but you can still play the tune'. Another reported her doctor called her uterus 'rubbish'.

Women's health groups objected to a pamphlet called *Curing*

17

the Hysterectomy Hang-ups used until very recently at National Women's Hospital and still used in some local hospitals. In it, Professor Dennis Bonham, head of the postgraduate school of obstetrics and gynaecology, said: 'All that you lose is something the size of a flattened pear.' Removing the womb, he said, was 'tak[ing] away the carrycot, not the playpen'. Women who were disturbed after the operation were disturbed before it, he maintained. 'Any ordinary person who isn't a psychiatric cripple will be perfectly all right.'

Unfortunately, this kind of blasé attitude to hysterectomy appears to have been influential. Such thinking is behind the use of hysterectomy as a method of sterilisation, rather than the simpler, less risky tubal ligation. This practice was not uncommon in New Zealand and elsewhere in the late seventies and early eighties. There has been a tendency to suggest hysterectomy for a wide variety of problems, even ones not necessarily cured by removal of the uterus, and to down-play the risks and problems. Women answering our questionnaire commonly told of doctors who said a hysterectomy would make them feel like 'a new woman', a somewhat emotive and manipulative way of talking about a major surgical procedure.

When women express their feelings about losing their uterus, they can be met with disbelief or dismissal. One woman (36 years old, three children) wrote of entering hospital in 1987 for a repair of the pelvic ligaments. She had been adamant beforehand that she would not have a hysterectomy. However, on admission she was told her prolapse was so bad she should have a hysterectomy.

> I said I wanted my womb. It was the centre of my body, all my energy channelled through there. He [the consultant] questioned it and I told him further, sexually it was very important to me. He said, No it isn't, you don't feel it during sex. I asked him how he knew, he was a man. We had this kind of talk for ages. He sent various other people to convince me it would be a good decision. At one point he told me to leave the hospital, get dressed and go home.

Finally the woman agreed to the hysterectomy and had an uneventful recovery, physically.

> Afterwards everybody was telling me how well I looked and how glad I'd be that I had made that decision. The specialist looked so pleased with himself. When they asked me how I felt, I just said OK because how I was really feeling was too devastating. I felt totally cheated at the short notice I was given to have the hysterectomy. That day I was in a highly emotional state. Now that it's gone, I can't replace it. I feel empty, ungrounded, off balance, decentralised, lower sexual energy, low capacity for orgasm ¯ .ish I'd stuck to my guns and not let them do it.

Liz McConville of the Christchurch Patients' Rights group told the *Sunday Times* in 1983 of experiences women had had in Christchurch.

> We have had cases where women who go to hospital [to have] certain things done have their uterus removed as well. And if they complain, they say: 'See, you are an emotional woman.' Women often allow themselves to be manipulated by doctors into having a hysterectomy. The surgery is the doctors' ground and women tended to go along with what doctors said, unless they were particularly assertive.

Women who answered our questionnaire gave examples of this rather casual attitude to removal of the womb. One woman who entered hospital in 1981 (50 years old, five children) for a prolapse operation was not told until five days later that her womb had also been removed during surgery.

> I asked the specialist how the operation had gone. After a slight hesitation he told me that it had gone well, but he had removed my womb because 'it was misshapen and no further use'. He said as it would save him having to get me in again, he thought it better to take it now. His statement was like a body blow. I felt devastated and then I realised why I was recovering so slowly. My body knew it had had a shock, even if I didn't. I felt as if he might

just as well have taken my heart out, and here he was calmly telling me, as if he had just pulled a carrot out of the garden. I was very upset afterwards . . . Subsequent testing proved nothing wrong with the womb.

This woman said she still mourned the loss of her womb and was easily upset over 'maternal issues'.

Personally I have always felt akin to a castrated animal. Happy — but no sex drive. This loss took a long time to come to terms with . . . I still get very angry at articles which imply that women who have problems like mine cause them through their own attitudes.

Another woman (43 years old, no children) entered hospital in 1963 for surgery for suspected bowel cancer. During the surgery 24 non-malignant growths were found on her reproductive organs, so all her organs were removed.

I had no mention of such an operation earlier as I had a small fibroid removed 18 months earlier and had been given a clean bill of health. The house surgeon told me in a matter-of-face way: 'We thought in view of your age it was just as well to remove the organs as well as the growths.' At that time I was full of morphine and didn't react very quickly. When my mind took it in, I wept and wept . . . I had never had children because of my husband's war injuries, but still felt totally devastated when I was speyed without any requests or questions. I still feel this to this day.

One woman experienced intense hot flushes, depression, loss of sexual interest and asthmatic attacks after the surgery but received no help. 'I went to see my GP who remarked "I don't know what you expect me to do." . . . My GP later said he wasn't aware my ovaries had been removed.'

Women occasionally reported the removal of other organs during the hysterectomy operation without prior discussion or permission. The ovaries were sometimes removed, even when healthy, and the appendix, sometimes for no reason at all.

All in the mind?

When women have reported negative effects of hysterectomy, such as feeling depressed or less like sex, these have often been dismissed as all in their minds. Although some New Zealand doctors do accept that removal of the womb can cause such problems, many deny it is possible. Because they have a view of the womb as simply a place to incubate babies, they cannot accept that its removal could influence other body organs. Therefore, when women report effects, it has to be all in their minds. This is not the view in many overseas countries. Research does exist that backs up women's experiences with negative after-effects, but unfortunately many New Zealand doctors have not kept themselves up-to-date with overseas thinking, even in the major teaching hospitals.

Throughout gynaecology in general, there has been a tendency to depict women as over-emotional, anxious and irrational and this can seriously interfere with the woman's ability to be heard, and to establish an equal relationship with her doctor. Problems in the pelvis, such as pain or heavy bleeding, are commonly put down to psychological causes or marital problems. If the doctor can find no organic cause, then we must have made it up or be exaggerating. Even asking questions is sometimes labelled as over-anxious.

One respondent to our questionnaire described how her doctor's attitude towards women got in the way of a proper investigation of her problem.

> My GP (a woman) diagnosed my tiredness and weakness as lack of exercise and neuroses for two years before bothering to test for anything. I was extremely anaemic with a haemoglobin level of 80 instead of the normal 160 when it was eventually picked up. The cause was one very large fibroid which caused the uterus to be as large as a 24-week pregnancy.

One writer in the *American Journal of Obstetrics and Gynaecology* on 'the post-hysterectomy problem patient' graphically illustrated the kind of stereotyped and plain silly thinking women encounter in some doctors. She blamed unnecessary hysterectomies on women whose symptoms were 'primarily neurotic'. She described three types of 'typical candidates for postoperative depression'. The first was the 'polysurgery addict', a 'hysterical neurotic' who repeatedly undergoes surgery because of 'a need to suffer'. The second was 'the indifferent woman' who immaturely refuses to think about the operation beforehand, but then has an 'uncontrolled, infantile response to postoperative discomforts'. And the third was the 'over-anxious woman who worries about everything from the site and size of the incision to the type of anaesthesia'.

Thus, a quite normal, healthy desire to know the facts becomes evidence of neurosis. In this view, the 'normal' woman patient is passive, accepting and uncomplaining. She also needs to be able to strike a balance between asking enough questions to avoid being 'immature' and asking so many as to be deemed 'over-anxious'!

Recently some doctors have begun to explain our high hysterectomy rate as a result of patient 'demand'. In March 1988 Dr Lorraine Welch of Wellington Women's Hospital argued in the *Evening Post* that it was explained by New Zealand doctors' allowing patients to be part of decision-making.

> There is a greater tendency by doctors here that if a problem such as heavy or painful periods is significant to her, and she wants to have a hysterectomy, then that is what she should have. It is hard for anyone else to judge how painful a woman's period may be or how frustrating constant, heavy periods are.

On the subject of patient 'demand', Margaret Ryan, who conducted a prospective study of women having hysterectomies in Melbourne, concluded: 'The data from this study does not present a woman as demanding, if anything it indicates patience and stoicism. For some the recommendation for surgery was a vindication that their symptoms were real and not the figment of neurotic imagination.'

Doctors have been defensive about criticisms of hysterectomy rates and, in the eighties, gynaecological teachers and some doctors are more aware that women's attitudes towards their bodies are complex, and that we do not all regard our wombs as simply a place to incubate babies, or our periods as something to be got rid of once we've had our children. However, they still sometimes fail to see that each woman is an individual who will have her own unique feelings about her body. Thus some doctors have swung around to a position that wombs must be preserved at all costs and menstruation is vitally important to us. Consequently, doctors experimenting with using the laser to destroy the endometrium as an alternative to hysterectomy in women with menorrhagia decided to leave a portion intact, so that menstruation would continue, even though the woman was sterile. They have overlooked the possibility that some women may be glad to have no periods.

We still have some distance to go before all doctors see women as individuals. No two women are the same and we will all have our own attitudes to our wombs.

Changing practices

We have some suggestions about ways of tackling New Zealand's high hysterectomy rate. Firstly, hospitals need to develop treatment protocols on hysterectomy. A protocol is a consensus statement, which should be worked out by doctors and consumers, giving agreed upon indications for the operation and how the patient should be managed. Consumers should have access to such a protocol that will guide them in their decision-making. This would protect women from being taken in by an individual doctor's unorthodox, overly zealous or out-of-date opinions.

Another strategy would be similar to that adopted in Saskatchewan, where there had been a dramatic increase in hysterectomies through the 1960s. At the request of the Saskatchewan Department of Health, a provincial medical association organised a committee of medical and non-medical people to look at the problem. The committee drafted a list of acceptable indications for hysterectomy, condemning 'sterilising, prophylactic, or birthday' hysterectomies. It surveyed major provincial hospitals and found the number of unnecessary hysterectomies ranged from 59 percent to 17 percent. There were no penalties for doctors who operated for reasons other than those listed, but the effect of this scrutiny was a decline in unnecessary hysterectomies to 7.8 percent in 1974. To encourage compliance the medical association met with administrators and staff in hospitals with high rates.

In California, legislation came into effect in 1988 requiring doctors to explain the possible risks and complications of hysterectomy, length of hospital stay, recovery time, costs and alternatives to hysterectomy. Written consent to hysterectomy was required by law. It is too early to say whether this kind of intervention will lead to a decrease in hysterectomy rates. In New Zealand, there is a plan to introduce consent forms which require the doctor to list the information she or he has given the woman. It would also list any other procedures the woman has agreed to. This more formal consent procedure could lead to more informed decision-making, but there is considerable opposition from the medical profession to such consent forms.

Unnecessary hysterectomies are a political issue, especially at a time of increasing stringency in health budgets. Governments possibly need to take a lead, to encourage health boards and professionals to re-evaluate their practices.

4

REASONS HYSTERECTOMY IS SUGGESTED

Our questionnaire asked women to indicate why they had had a hysterectomy, and gave a checklist of 10 possible reasons. The largest group (72 percent) gave heavy bleeding as a reason, although, because several boxes could be ticked, this was usually combined with another reason. In 33 percent of cases it was combined with fibroids.

A survey of all hysterectomies in the United States over a 15-year period showed that 10.7 percent were performed for cancer and carcinoma in situ of the cervix, 26 percent for fibroids, 14 percent for endometriosis, 20 percent for prolapse, 6 percent for endometrial hyperplasia and 20 percent for 'other', which included bleeding without a diagnosis of disease.

Hysterectomies are suggested in several situations: when there is a disease that can be diagnosed, such as cancer or endometriosis, when there is a malfunction or 'disorder' of the uterus for which no definite cause can be found, or where there has been accidental damage to the uterus. Professor John Hutton of the Wellington Clinical School says that at Wellington Women's Hospital about 50 percent of hysterectomies are performed for an organic disease and the other 50 percent for heavy bleeding of uncertain cause.

Cancer is one situation where there will be a fairly cut and dried recommendation of hysterectomy. The operation will probably be life saving because not to have it means the disease may progress to a terminal stage. There are still decisions to be made, but most women will agree without demur to a hysterectomy for cancer.

For the other diseases and disorders there may be a choice between hysterectomy and other therapies, or simply doing nothing, as menopause will often provide a cure. To make an informed decision it is important to have information about the complaint and the likelihood that hysterectomy will cure or at least alleviate it. Other options need to be considered.

Women need to be aware that hysterectomy is sometimes suggested as a 'cure' for disorders that will probably not be helped by the removal of the uterus. One woman who answered our questionnaire wrote that the operation did nothing for her repeated bladder infections, the reason she was advised to have it. 'Nine years later I still get them and the operation has produced side effects such as discomfort after intercourse which I certainly never had previously.'

Another described having a hysterectomy for back pain. 'At the time I was willing to accept any advice that would bring relief for my back problem. However, the hysterectomy didn't help at all. I felt it just added insult to injury.' Ultimately, she needed major back surgery. 'I do wonder,' she wrote, 'if a 43-year-old male had back problems, would any male doctor suggest he be sterilised?'

The most common disorders leading to hysterectomy are menstrual pain and excessive bleeding. Both can be caused by disease, for example endometriosis will cause both pain and excess bleeding, and fibroids can cause heavy painful periods, but sometimes the doctor can come up with no specific condition to explain these symptoms.

Disorders

Excessive bleeding

Normal periods occur every 28 days and last for 4 or 5 days. Bleeding of more than seven days is uncommon and experienced by only 1–2 percent of women. A normal cycle is between 25 and 32 days. A short cycle and long period means, of course, that the woman has far fewer bleeding-free days. She can feel as if she constantly has her period.

Heavy bleeding is a frequent reason given for advising a hysterectomy. The doctor cannot find a treatable cause and the heavy periods are making the woman's life miserable. There are differences in what women will tolerate in their menstrual flow, but it is clear that some women endure years of debilitating periods, which might have been ended by a hysterectomy. These women frequently report that they feel totally rejuvenated after the operation.

Sometimes the menstrual flow becomes so heavy that the woman is constantly soaking through pads. She may need to wear two tampons and a pad and still have 'accidents'. Some women become housebound during their period and cannot even go to the bank or shops, let alone go to work. In the worst cases they resort to plastic pants, babies' nappies or simply sitting on the lavatory for part of the day. They are constantly washing clothes and bed linen and are not able to contemplate sex for quite some days a month.

Anaemia is a frequent result of such heavy bleeding so that iron tablets or injections are necessary, but the woman still feels constantly tired. Women were probably able to cope better with heavy bleeding in the days when married women did not go out to work; constant trips to the lavatory, 'accidents' and cleaning oneself up are more difficult in the workplace.

One woman whose doctor initially refused her request for hysterectomy on the grounds she was too young (she was 33, mother of three children) wrote that her bleeding got worse and worse as she got older.

> I was wearing internal and external pads plus as much towelling as I could fit inside my pants. Even then, I could only be away from the house for an hour at a time or be with sympathetic

friends who understood if I made a dash for the nearest private place (often the seat of a car) to change all my padding.

The final straw came when despite her precautions blood ran down into her shoes in the street. She got to her car and drove home.

> [I] spent a full eight minutes on the toilet, cleaned myself up, had a good cry, then set out for the bank again. While standing in the queue, the same thing happened again. I went home and rang for an appointment with my doctor. I went to see him and allowed myself the luxury of mild hysterics, saying that if he didn't recommend me for a hysterectomy, I was going to do the job myself. He frowned, but didn't ridicule me. At the hospital they said I should have been there years ago.

Two days after the operation, she reported she was 'dancing down the ward to meet my doctor, carrying all the operation paraphernalia . . . He was smiling at my youthful exuberance and saying "Be careful or the rest will drop out." '

There has been a tendency for doctors to discount heavy bleeding and think that women are exaggerating or complaining too much. But heavy bleeding should always be investigated because it could signal a serious disease such as cancer or a progressively debilitating one, such as pelvic inflammatory disease or endometriosis.

Some women bleed a lot because their blood doesn't coagulate very effectively. A coagulation screen may show that their coagulation system isn't very efficient. There may be a family history of bleeding or bruising easily. If the test is normal, the cause of the bleeding may be either a failure of the muscles in the uterus to contract the small blood vessels, or it will be hormonal.

Too much oestrogen can make the endometrial lining grow thicker and periods heavier and longer; too little progesterone can cause the endometrium to be thin and come away earlier, resulting in frequent, prolonged periods. Your doctor might prescribe some combination of these hormones, such as oral contraceptives, or progesterone alone, to see if these control the bleeding before a hysterectomy is contemplated. Danazol, used in the treatment of endometriosis, is prescribed by some doctors. See the section on endometriosis (p. 38) for further information on this drug. Bear in mind that being underweight or overweight can have an effect on hormones, so attaining the right weight could result in an improvement in menstruation.

Women who experience heavy bleeding with an IUD in place should have it removed because this frequently instantly results in a 'cure'.

As we get older, our periods may change. In our late thirties and forties they can become heavier, with more clots. Some women have episodes of 'flooding' in the years before and during menopause, which can be a very alarming experience. In this age group we are also less likely to be relying on hormonal methods of contraception, which had the advantage of cutting down bleeding, and more likely to be using male or female sterilisation as birth control. Our real cycles are thus not masked by hormones.

A dilatation and curettage is usually recommended for heavy bleeding because it can diagnose any disease that may be present, check for cancer and may cure the bleeding. It's not clear exactly how a D & C can stop heavy periods. Sometimes a second D & C will cure heavy bleeding where an initial one failed, but there's no point in having repeated D & Cs if there has been no improvement after a second one. One woman responding to our questionnaire reported having had five D & Cs performed privately for heavy bleeding 'until we finally came to the stunned conclusion that the consultant was doing them for financial gain'.

Herbal remedies, diet and exercise may be helpful in reducing the menstrual flow and pain. Avoid red meats, eggs, fatty foods and excess dairy foods (but keep your calcium intake up). Eliminate alcohol and smoking. A good naturopath or herbalist could suggest suitable remedies, but of the herbs, raspberry leaf tea, comfrey and red clover are noted for their kindly influence on the uterus. Homoeopathy, yoga and acupuncture are other avenues to explore. For a list of registered natural healers (such as naturopaths, homoeopaths and herbalists) in your area, write to the Register of Natural Therapists, PO Box 11-311, Auckland.

Menstrual pain

Very painful periods is another disorder that sometimes leads to hysterectomy. Although diseases such as endometriosis cause period pain, sometimes no disease cause can be found. Menstrual pain is much more frequently found in the young, and it usually decreases with age. Menstrual pain may also improve if women use the Pill as contraception.

One woman who answered our questionnaire had a hysterectomy at 29 for extreme menstrual pain, ending years of crippling pain. She wrote: 'From the age of 11 I have had painful periods with vomiting and diarrhoea and 2 days off school and work each month.' Oral contraceptives and childbirth made no difference to the pain. When she answered the questionnaire it was only 10 weeks after her hysterectomy, but she reported a positive outcome. 'My hair is healthy and shiny, my skin is great and my eyes are sparkly, so after all these years I feel wonderful and know I made the right decision.'

There are things that women can do to try and diminish menstrual pain. Some factors in our lifestyles may contribute to the pain. Smoking increases pain as nicotine increases muscle activity in the uterus and stress and tension can increase pain. It is possible to learn from a therapist techniques for coping with and alleviating pain. Hypnosis, acupuncture, acupressure, yoga, anti-spasmodic drugs, orgasm through sex with partner or masturbation, and body massage may relieve menstrual pain. A study published in *Obstetrics and Gynaecology* in 1987 showed that 90 percent of women who had weekly acupuncture for painful periods showed improvement, with a 41 percent reduction in the use of painkillers.

Some menstrual cramps are caused by hormones called

prostaglandins, which stimulate the uterus during menstruation and childbirth. Anti-prostaglandin drugs such as mefenamic acid (Ponstan) block the release of prostaglandins. They usually reduce menstrual bleeding to about half and as they have few side-effects can be used for long periods of time.

Overseas, some doctors are using diathermy (burning) or laser treatment to destroy the endometrium, but leave the uterus intact. The woman is of course sterile, but avoids the major surgery of hysterectomy. This will soon be available in parts of New Zealand.

Diseases

Fibroids

Fibroids are one of the most common causes of an enlarged uterus and one of the most common causes of hysterectomy. They are benign growths or tumours of the uterus. They grow in the thick muscular wall of the uterus and may be the size of a pea or much bigger than a grapefruit. In themselves they are harmless, but they can cause pain and excessive menstrual bleeding. It is most unlikely that a suspected fibroid will be malignant. Fewer than 0.2 percent are ever found to be malignant. It is disturbing that a number of women filling out our questionnaire agreed to a hysterectomy because they said they were told their fibroids could be malignant. In the absence of any proof, this amounts to scaring women into hysterectomy, for the possibility of cancer is extremely remote.

Fibroids are very common: about one-quarter of women over 30 has one or more of these growths, and they are not always treated. Most women are unaware they even have them. They can, however, grow larger as we get older and cause increased pain and heavier bleeding during menstruation. Heavy blood loss can lead to anaemia and a continual feeling of tiredness and weakness. The growth of fibroids is probably promoted by the hormone

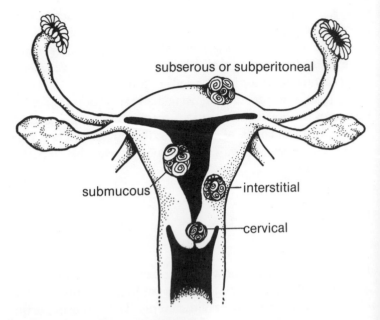

Various types of uterine fibroids.

oestrogen, so after menopause, when the ovaries produce less oestrogen they usually stop growing or shrink and give no trouble. Women with problems caused by fibroids need to weigh up whether they wish to remove the uterus containing the growths to end the problem, or hang on until menopause in the knowledge that the problem will end there.

Because oestrogen probably promotes growth, women with fibroids should avoid oral contraceptives containing oestrogen, and oestrogen replacement therapy during menopause. Fibroids already present may increase in size during pregnancy when oestrogen levels are raised. Some women have children despite the presence of fibroids, but there can be problems. Conception can be difficult because of the growth inside the uterus and a large fibroid can leave the foetus insufficient room to grow, leading to premature labour. Occasionally a Caesarian section will be necessary because the cervical passage is blocked by the growth.

Fibroids can grow in different parts of the uterus and their location determines any problems they might cause. The most common sort, called interstitial fibroids, are confined in the uterine wall. If they grow towards the outside wall of the uterus they are called subserous or subperitoneal fibroids. If they grow towards the inside wall they are called submucous fibroids. Fibroids in the cervix are called cervical fibroids.

Although occasionally a woman may become aware of a fibroid if it becomes very large and causes a pot belly or protuberance in the abdomen, it is usually detected by a doctor during a vaginal examination. Because some fibroids that grow out from the outside wall of the uterus can be confused with ovarian growths, ultrasound may be used to distinguish the two.

Submucous fibroids can be difficult to feel by a vaginal examination, but during a D & C the doctor can feel the bulge with the curette while scraping the inside walls of the uterus. A special X-ray called a hysterosalpingogram sometimes shows up a submucous fibroid.

Subserous fibroids can grow outwards, remaining attached to the uterus by a stalk or stem. If the stalk is long and thin, it can twist causing acute pain. The fibroid's blood supply can be cut off causing it to 'die', resulting in more pain. These pendunculated fibroids can also put pressure on the bladder if they are near it, leading to pain and more frequent urination, or the bowel, causing pain or difficulty in passing a motion. Cervical fibroids can also cause bladder problems. Cervical fibroids can distort the cervix or protrude into the vagina.

Occasionally a submucous fibroid will fill the interior cavity of the uterus and the uterus will react by trying to push it out, especially during menstruation. These contractions can be very painful and usually continue throughout the menstrual period. Occasionally they can become pendunculated and protrude through the cervix, and these are called fibroid polyps. They may become infected or bleed.

Submucous fibroids sometimes produce heavy periods with large clots because they increase the surface area of the endometrium and distort it. The periods may become longer, with the time between periods shorter. If there is infection or the fibroid dies, there may be a bad-smelling discharge.

Fibroids increase menstrual bleeding by interfering with the blood supply, attracting blood to the pelvis by a system we as yet do not understand.

Pain can be caused at times other than menstruation. Interstitial fibroids can caused a dull ache in the lower abdomen. Adhesions or scar tissue may build up around the fibroid, fixing the uterus to other organs and this can cause back, abdominal or menstrual pain and occasionally pain during intercourse. Fibroids pressing on other organs can cause discomfort, especially if you stand for a long time. This pain is felt in the back, abdomen and inside of the thighs. Pressure on veins can cause varicose veins or piles.

If the fibroids are small and not producing troublesome symptoms, most doctors will advise doing nothing in the expectation that the fibroids will regress after menopause. If the fibroid is very large and/or causing severe symptoms, the wait-and-see approach is not sensible. Later complications are possible if large fibroids are not removed.

Treatment is usually hysterectomy. Occasionally a pendunculated submucous fibroid, a protruding submucous fibroid or a cervical fibroid can be removed by a D & C.

If the woman is young and wants to have more children, she may be offered a myomectomy. This surgery cuts out the fibroids but leaves the uterus intact. After the operation a woman has about a 50 percent chance of getting pregnant. This is a difficult operation with a higher complication rate than hysterectomy and for this reason it is not often performed. The uterus bleeds easily, and if this cannot be controlled during the operation a hysterectomy may have to be performed. There can be many post-operative complications and there is also the possibility the fibroids will come back. Adhesions can form leading to pain on intercourse, backache and abnormal bleeding. Success depends on the size and position of the fibroids.

In America some doctors are inclining more towards removal of the fibroids only using laser surgery, retaining the uterus. They report successes with this approach, which also cuts down bleeding during surgery. Patient demand in New Zealand could pressure doctors to consider this or other alternatives. Because hysterectomy is commonplace and doctors have become quite expert at doing it, they may not themselves be motivated to think creatively about alternative treatments.

Birth control pills are sometimes recommended, but while these may curb menstrual bleeding, they may make the fibroid increase in size, leading to the need for hysterectomy. Oestrogen replacement therapy after menopause could also increase the size of the fibroids. Women should think carefully, and obtain a second opinion before undertaking these treatments.

There is no readily available drug treatment for fibroids. Some drugs have been developed, but they are currently too expensive for general use.

Pelvic inflammatory disease

Pelvic inflammatory disease (PID) is persistent infection in the pelvic organs. In some women it can be a chronic low-grade infection causing a feeling of lethargy and of being constantly unwell. Other women have recurrent acute attacks.

Doctors sometimes have difficulty diagnosing PID, especially the chronic low-grade variety. Women reporting symptoms of vague pelvic pain, painful sexual intercourse and tiredness may be classed 'malingering' women who invent pelvic symptoms because of dissatisfactions about other areas of their lives. Some doctors prescribe tranquillisers for these symptoms and the woman does not get the treatment she needs. The woman might get tired of constantly visiting the doctor and being disbelieved and so stop going. Her confidence might be knocked by her doctor's attitude and her failure to find the cause of her symptoms. There might be judgemental comments about her own or her husband's sexual habits, which can cause suspicion between the man and woman because PID is sometimes caused by a sexually transmitted disease. PID can be the result of gonorrhoea or chlamydia, and if this is the case the husband also must be treated. There are, however, other causes of PID, and non-gonococcal PID is generally more serious in its effects. PID can be caused by bacteria or organisms harmless when found on other parts of the body, but lethal in the normally sterile uterus. Infection from an operation such as appendectomy, or from childbirth, miscarriage or abortion, can develop into PID. We also now know that users of intra-uterine devices can develop PID, especially users of plastic IUDs left in place for many years. No woman should be now using a plastic IUD, for example, Saf-T-Coil, Lippes Loop and Dalkon Shields. PID can also develop with copper IUDs, and any woman who has an infection with an IUD in place should insist on having the IUD removed as well an antibiotic treatment. She should not use an IUD again.

The symptoms of pelvic infection are:

- A change in the flow and length of menstrual periods
- Increased pain during periods
- Bleeding or spotting at other times
- Pelvic pain
- Pain during or after intercourse
- A smelly discharge
- Fever or chills
- Tiredness and/or nausea
- Lower back pain
- Burning and frequency of urination
- Swollen abdomen
- Bowel problems such as constipation.

A woman may have all, some or none of these symptoms.

Infection can usually be diagnosed by testing swabs taken from the vagina. Sometimes a laparoscopy will be performed. This is a small operation to look at the pelvic organs and see if there is active infection or scar tissue caused by repeated infection. Auckland gynaecologist Paul Hutchison believes that if PID is suspected but not proven on two occasions, a laparoscopy is advisable.

Untreated or wrongly treated infection in the womb will spread up the Fallopian tubes and into the pelvic cavity to other organs such as the ovaries. It can lead to peritonitis and be life-threatening. The body tries to deal with the infection by sealing it off with scar tissue and this can 'glue' body organs together. The infection can become inaccessible to drug treatment and never be fully cured. The PID sufferer may become infertile or experience ectopic pregnancy because the tubes are blocked.

Treatment for PID is with antibiotics, which in acute episodes will be given intravenously in hospital. Sometimes attempts are made to remove adhesions surgically and separate pelvic organs, but the success rate is not high. Many women find they still have pelvic pain after the operation. Some women have found long-term acupuncture helpful for the pain of PID and good diet, exercise, rest and avoidance of stress may help limit attacks.

Occasionally a woman with a severe acute attack will need to have an emergency hysterectomy, and other women with incurable PID may ultimately choose to have a hysterectomy. The alternative is chronic pelvic pain. Professor Colin Mantell describes hysterectomy as 'the end of the road treatment' for infection, while at Wellington Women's Hospital, Professor John Hutton says hysterectomies are rarely performed for this reason.

The uterus and tubes would be removed, and the ovaries conserved if possible. However, the ovaries can become abscessed and may have to be removed. A hysterectomy for PID would almost certainly be performed abdominally so the doctor can inspect the tubes and ovaries for infection and remove them if necessary. Professor Mantell says that more than 80 percent of women who have hysterectomies for PID obtain freedom from pain. However, if the PID has damaged organs such as the bowel, the woman may continue to have some problems.

One of the women who responded to our questionnaire had a hysterectomy at 48 for repeated pelvic infection. She had suffered 7 years of PID with 12 hospital admissions in this time. Since her hysterectomy in 1985 she has been free of infection and of pain.

Endometriosis

This painful disease occurs when clumps of endometrial-like cells grow in the wrong place. They grow on the ovaries or tubes, the outside of the uterus or inside the pelvic cavity. Pieces of endometrium can also invade the ligaments supporting the uterus and between the uterus and bowel. This tissue behaves just like the endometrial lining of the uterus and bleeds each month. Because the blood has nowhere to go, 'chocolate cysts' develop and these cause pain and other problems. Chocolate cysts can be as tiny as a pinhead or quite large. If they break, they spread endometrial tissue through the pelvic cavity. Scar tissue and adhesions form, again causing pain, and the endometriosis can spread to the bowel, bladder and vagina, causing further problems in those parts of the body.

The main symptom of endometriosis is pain, although about 25 percent of afflicted women have no pain. The pelvic organs can become stuck together so that movement of the cervix during intercourse, vaginal examination by a doctor or normal movement may be very painful. Constipation and pain on moving the bowels, pain on urination and other bladder disturbances are common, but pain during menstruation is the telltale sign. It is dull and steady rather than cramp-like and becomes worse with each period. The amount of pain is not necessarily related to the extent of the disease. Abnormal menstrual bleeding, fatigue, depression, back pain and infertility (in about 40 percent of cases) are other effects of endometriosis. In one survey of women with endometriosis, 60 percent said they were unable to carry out normal tasks sometimes for several days each month, or for months and even years.

A doctor may diagnose endometriosis from feeling it as knobbly growths during a bimanual vaginal examination, but often a laparoscopic examination is necessary to see the cysts.

There are drug treatments for endometriosis, but these can have severe side-effects, and there might be disagreement between doctors about the most appropriate drug for an individual woman. For older women, a wait-and-see approach and painkillers in the meantime may be suggested, because the bleeding will stop at menopause. Women who want children may decide to delay treatment until they have a family. They will usually be advised not to delay too long before getting pregnant because of the infertility risk. During pregnancy endometriosis regresses in some women because there is no menstruation. If endometriosis is extensive, treatment is necessary because a ruptured ovarian cyst could mean emergency surgery.

The various drug treatments have one thing in common: they stop ovulation and prevent menstruation. Stopping periods can sometimes result in a cure. The most common drug is Danazol, a derivative of the male hormone testosterone, but some women find Danazol treament traumatic, especially because many of the side-effects are masculinising. It can cause excessive weight gain, bloating, nausea, depression, facial and chest hair, deepening of the voice and enlargement of the clitoris. Since Danazol induces a state not unlike the menopause, menopause-like symptoms are not uncommon, for example, hot flushes, vaginal dryness and vulvitis. A lower dose will reduce the side-effects. Danazol is usually given for a term of six to nine months, but even when treatment stops some of the masculinising effects, such as the lowering of the voice, may not go away.

Another hormone treatment is Provera, which contains progesterone and is similar to Depo Provera. It carries the same risks as Depo Provera — weight gain, depression, loss of libido, unknown long-term cancer risk — and may affect future fertility. Norithisterone, another progesterone, is also used.

In mild cases, oral contraceptives may be prescribed as these prevent ovulation and cut down menstrual bleeding. However, the dose may need to be increased to several pills a day and this will markedly increase any hormone-induced side-effects. This kind of treatment will control, not cure, the disease and is not often used nowadays.

No hormone treatment is 100 percent effective. About 30–40 percent of women using Danazol will have a recurrence of endometriosis within three years. Hormone treatment is not effective in cases where there is enlargement of the ovaries.

Conservative surgery involves attempting to remove all the chocolate cysts by surgery or diathermy (burning) and to separate adhesions. However, the surgery itself may cause adhesions and the disease does recur in a significant number of cases. For a woman who wants children, however, it could give her the time to begin a family.

If the disease is extensive or the woman has a completed family, more extensive surgery, for example, hysterectomy, may be suggested as a last resort. If the uterus is removed, often the tubes and ovaries are removed as well because the ovaries produce the hormones that aggravate the disease. In younger women, retaining the ovaries, if at all possible, is favoured. If the ovaries are removed and oestrogen replacement therapy given, the oestrogen would affect any areas of endometriosis that haven't been removed. As well as removing the major organs the doctor would try to remove all the nodules of endometriosis. Sometimes there can be over 25 of these. Whatever your age, you would have to think carefully before agreeing to removal of your ovaries.

One of the respondents to our questionnaire had unsuccessful treatment by hysterectomy for endometriosis. She had endometriosis for 17 years before it was diagnosed. 'I was told I was mad in the head and to pull myself together. After going from doctor to doctor I had a hysterectomy when I was 32.' For two months after the hysterectomy in 1979, she felt well, but since then the endometriosis has spread. She is now showing some improvement with progesterone tablets.

The recurrence rate after hysterectomy, whether or not the ovaries are removed, is very low. If it does come back, Danazol or further surgery would be options. A special laser is being used with some success overseas and will soon be offered in parts of New Zealand.

Adenomyosis

Adenomyosis is a kind of internal endometriosis, in which endometrial tissue invades the uterus. The uterus becomes enlarged and bulky, with sometimes heavy, painful periods. Up to 40 percent of women with this condition suffer no symptoms at all; around 20 percent will, however, suffer severely. There is no really accurate way of diagnosing this disease and it is usually only discovered when the pathologist examines the uterus after a hysterectomy for heavy, painful periods.

Pelvic relaxation and prolapse

Sometimes wear and tear, especially caused by pregnancy and childbirth, can cause the muscles supporting the uterus and the upper walls of the vagina to become weak and slack. The walls of the vagina then sag inwards under the weight of the urethra, the bladder and the rectum. You might find that sneezing, jumping or running causes urine to leak out. This only happens when you are upright, showing that the problem is primarily one of lack of pelvic support. This is called stress incontinence.

Sometimes the weak muscles become so stretched and thin they begin to separate and tear, and the urethra, bladder or rectum can bulge into the vagina. This can usually be felt as a lump or bulge in the vaginal wall. These conditions are called urethrocele (urethra), cystocele (bladder) and rectocele (rectum). A rectocele may be unnoticed or may cause constipation. A cystocele can make it difficult to completely empty the bladder and thus cause recurrent bladder infections because the bladder never empties properly. A chronically irritated bladder floor can cause urge incontinence, the sudden loss of drops of urine. It is

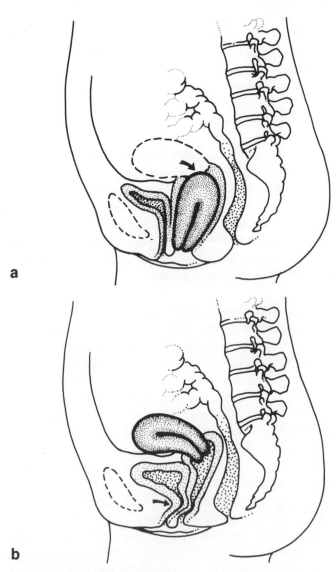

Various types of prolapse.

a. *Prolapse of the uterus. The uterus has dropped down into the vagina. The drawing shows a second degree prolapse.*

b. *Urethrocele. The urethra bulges into the vagina.*

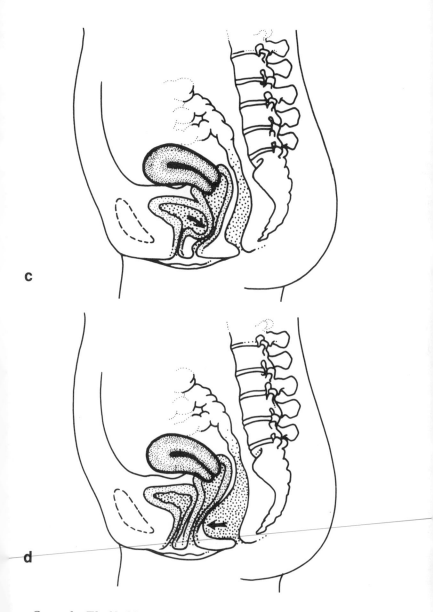

c

d

c. *Cystocele. The bladder wall bulges into the vagina.*
d. *Rectocele. The rectal wall bulges into the vagina.*

very important to distinguish between urge incontinence caused by a cystocele and urge incontinence caused by problems in the bladder itself before initiating treatment, because they call for different remedies.

Where loss of pelvic support is marked, the uterus can start to fall into the vagina and might be felt by the woman or her partner during sexual intercourse. The uterus can even drop so far into the vagina that it can be felt or seen at the vaginal entrance. This is called prolapse. Women with any of these conditions might suffer a heavy, dragging feeling in the pelvic area, as if everything is going to drop out, particularly when they stand for a long time.

Prolapse was once quite common because women had little help with difficult labours and pushed for far too long, or they had too many children too close together because they did not have effective contraception. Happily, prolapse happens less frequently today. Prolapse can occur in overweight women, women who cough frequently because of a lung condition and chronically constipated women who strain when going to the lavatory. Age is also a major factor and the withdrawal of oestrogen at menopause can worsen a cystocele or rectocele problem.

In deciding what course of treatment to follow it is important to understand what organs have been affected and how severe the condition is. Make sure you are given a full explanation of what has happened in your vagina. Some doctors will recommend simply repairing the prolapse as long as it is not too severe, while others will argue that repair will be less successful if the uterus is not removed. Get a second or third opinion if your doctor suggests hysterectomy for mild prolapse.

In the early stages of pelvic relaxation, when the main symptoms are stress incontinence and weak vaginal walls, exercise can be helpful. The aim of Kegel's exercise is to strengthen the band of muscle that stretches like a hammock from the pubic bone in the front to the tail bone at the back and surrounds the urethra, vagina and rectum. The exercise is very simple, consisting of regularly tightening the muscle, but before starting you need to find the right muscle. This can be a bit difficult if it lacks strength. As you tighten the muscle you will feel a tightening sensation around the vulva and anus — some women describe it as a 'pulling up' or 'gathering' feeling. To make sure you have identified the right muscle, try stopping and starting the flow when urinating. The exercises can be done in any position — sitting, standing, lying or walking, or during sexual intercourse — and they must be done frequently, about 100–200 a day, each one held for 3 seconds.

You should notice an improvement in about two months. You should have more bladder control, and both you and your partner may notice an improvement in feeling during intercourse. Women with haemorrhoids (piles) might find they disappear.

Studies have shown that women who have been taught how to do these exercises by a specially trained physiotherapist have the most success. Most major obstetric and women's hospitals have such a person on the staff. Ask your doctor to find one for you. In Auckland the Incontinence Society can refer you to a qualified person.

If the relaxation has progressed to the extent of a marked cystocele or rectocele, the defects in the internal muscles can be repaired by taking a 'tuck' in the vagina. If you have a uterine prolapse that is not severe, a repair operation could be done. The stretched section is removed and the uterus lifted back into place.

Surgeons have their own ideas about what the vagina should be like and some think they are doing the woman, or more likely her husband, a favour by making the vagina 'tighter'. During the repair operation the surgeon may damage the vagina to make the repair more effective. Sexist stereotyping of older women can be a factor in the course of action a gynaecologist suggests.

At medical symposia, gynaecologists often make a distinction between 'young' and 'older' women, but they do not make clear where 'old' starts. They will decide that some procedures are best for 'young' women, while different criteria and methods will be used on 'older' women. 'Young' women are expected to be sexually attractive and active and loss of any function is seen as 'tragic'. 'Older' women are to some extent seen as sexually disqualified, and not interested in their sexual lives. It is not seen as a tragedy if the woman is surgically mutilated or disfigured.

You need to discuss with your doctor the subject of sexual intercourse and how you feel about your vagina. Even if you do not have a sexual partner at the time, or are celibate by choice, you might want to retain a 'whole' vagina to feel good about yourself as a woman. Imagine how a man would feel about his penis being disfigured, even if he had no lover. These are sometimes difficult things to talk about, but a gynaecologist who cannot listen and sympathise with how you feel is probably not a good person to be operating on your body.

For some women it may be possible to deal with a prolapse by using a Hodge pessary. This is a polythene ring, a bit like a contraceptive diaphragm, which can be inserted high in the vagina to hold the uterus in place. This can be a solution for elderly women for whom surgery might be a risk. However, a Hodge pessary can create problems: it can cause a smelly discharge, irritate the vagina and get in the way during intercourse. It must also be removed, cleaned and replaced every six to eight weeks and this requires a visit to the doctor.

Hormone replacement therapy is also sometimes tried for pelvic relaxation.

Hysterectomy should be reserved for women with severe prolapses who no longer want children. It should not be routinely performed when a vaginal cystocele or rectocele is repaired. After all, there is nothing wrong with the uterus itself, it is the supporting muscles that need repair. A hysterectomy for pelvic relaxation is usually performed vaginally because it also involves repair in the vagina.

Damage

Sterilisation and complications of contraception

Until very recently some gynaecologists performed hysterectomy as a method of sterilisation. They argued that as the uterus was a potential site for cancer and if the woman didn't 'need' her uterus any more, they would make her sterile by removing the uterus rather than tying her tubes. Fortunately, most gynaecologists have stopped thinking this way, but there are still some who use hysterectomy as a method of sterilisation.

There are compelling arguments against this practice. Sterilisation is a relatively simple operation, which can usually be performed by laparoscopy through a tiny incision in the abdomen. It has few known side-effects. Hysterectomy, however, is major surgery, with greater risks and longer recovery time. There can occasionally be long-term effects of hysterectomy, including effects on sexual response, which will not occur after a simple tubal ligation. If a doctor suggests hysterectomy to you as a method of sterilisation when your uterus is healthy, it would be important to seek a second opinion. Hysterectomy should never be used as a method of abortion, as has sometimes occurred in the past.

There is controversy over whether a woman who has a tubal ligation is more likely than an unsterilised woman to need a hysterectomy later on. Some research has shown that up to a third of women who have tubal ligations return for hysterectomies because of greatly increased bleeding. A 1987 Canadian study published in the *American Journal of Epidemiology* concluded that there were higher hysterectomy rates in women who had the tubal ligation when they were aged 25–29, but no increase in women who were sterilised when they were over 30. The study took a very large number of women who were matched to a control group for gynaecological disorders, including menstrual ones.

Because of the likelihood of hysterectomy following

sterilisation, some private health insurance companies will not pay for sterilisation done by tying the tubes, but will pay for sterilisation performed by hysterectomy: they argue that they would rather pay for one operation than two. This puts the woman in a very awkward position, as she should not be pressured to accept major surgery when a minor procedure would achieve what she wants. It is a subject that needs to be checked when taking out health insurance.

It is possible that a tubal ligation, in interrupting the blood supply between uterus and ovaries, causes changes in the normal functioning of these organs, leading to increased menstrual bleeding. Some studies have shown that the production of oestrogen from the ovaries decreases after tubal ligation.

Some doctors argue, however, that there are other reasons for the greater number of hysterectomies in women who have been sterilised. They point out that women who have been on hormonal contraception that inhibits menstruation will return to their 'natural' menstrual cycle once the sterilisation is performed. The Pill or Depo Provera may have disguised a normally heavy menstrual flow.

It's possible, too, that women who have been sterilised, who have made an active decision not to have more children, won't put up with difficult menstruation and may more readily seek action to end it.

At the moment we simply don't know whether sterilisation does in itself cause an increase in menstruation for some women, although the evidence that it does is accumulating. As a precaution, it would be a good idea to come off hormonal contraception six months before a planned sterilisation, to see what normal menstruation is like. An alternative is for the male partner to have a vasectomy, a very simple, effective procedure.

Occasionally, contraceptive problems can lead directly to hysterectomy. Women who use IUDs risk PID and hysterectomy in severe cases. Women using IUDs also risk hysterectomy through other causes. These are uncommon but women should be aware of them.

Occasionally during an IUD insertion, a perforation occurs. This happens when the device is pushed into or through the wall of the uterus. Very occasionally the perforation is so severe that emergency surgery must be performed, which could involve removing the uterus if it is bleeding uncontrollably. This can also occur as a severe complication of a D & C operation. A perforation or broken IUD will require surgery to locate the IUD or the pieces. If the IUD is easily located it can be surgically removed, but several New Zealand women have had hysterectomies in this situation and some have been successful in claims for injury to the Accident Compensation Corporation.

IUD use can also result in hysterectomy where menstruation becomes extremely heavy and remains that way after the removal of the IUD. The same thing can happen to users of Depo Provera. Women using Depo Provera usually have very scanty irregular bleeding, but in about 5 percent of users the bleeding becomes heavier and the periods longer. Doctors are not sure how to control this bleeding and usually try hormones or another shot of Depo Provera. Occasionally, if this is not successful, a hysterectomy might be performed. In America, a woman who had a hysterectomy after using Depo Provera recently won substantial damages from the drug's manufacturers.

Obstetric catastrophe and abortion emergency

Very rarely a hysterectomy may be performed to save a woman's life. Uncontrollable haemorrhage during an abortion is very rare, but sometimes the removal of the uterus is the only way of stopping the bleeding.

If the uterus ruptures during childbirth a hysterectomy would usually be performed to save the mother. A ruptured uterus might occur with prolonged, obstructed labour, especially if the woman has had a previous Caesarian section. A ruptured uterus is occasionally caused by the use of prostaglandins to speed up labour. Another emergency situation in childbirth is uncontrollable haemorrhage caused by a placenta that would not come away. Although an emergency Caesarian section is usually performed under these circumstances, a hysterectomy may occasionally be necessary.

5

GYNAECOLOGICAL CANCERS AND THEIR PRECURSORS

Although women can often exercise some choice about whether to have a hysterectomy or not, when we have cancer or some precancerous conditions our choices may be much more limited. It may be absolutely vital to have the hysterectomy or may increase the likelihood of a cure.

We need to be able to distinguish between cancer and its non-invasive precursors because they will usually call for different treatments and the risks will be quite different. It is easy to be scared by cancer. One doctor likened the mere mention of the word to 'waving the shroud'. Many of the cancer precursors, however, need relatively minor treatment, and will probably not involve hysterectomy. We have to remain clear-headed enough to decide on a sensible course of action without over-reacting.

For women who do have cancer it will be one of the most terrifying events in their lives. The treatment for many gynaecological cancers is harrowing and these women will need tremendous support: fortunately, the staff in most cancer wards are able to give this support. It is also possible for women and their families to call on the Cancer Society for help.

Endometrial hyperplasia
Hyperplasia means 'over-growth' and in this condition the lining of the uterus grows too thick. It is usually a benign condition,

occurring in women when their periods start or end. In older post-menopausal women it can sometimes be a precursor of endometrial cancer.

Endometrial hyperplasia is caused by continual oestrogen stimulation of the uterine lining, without the counterbalancing effect of progesterone, which makes the endometrium come away as a period. Oestrogen replacement therapy can cause this condition, but it can also occur in post-menopausal women not taking oestrogen and in young women. Polycystic ovarian disease can cause endometrial hyperplasia.

Irregular bleeding can be a sign of endometrial hyperplasia. At first the excess oestrogen stops menstrual bleeding, then as the endometrium builds up, pieces break up and come away. Eventually there can be quite profuse bleeding. A D & C or endometrial biopsy can diagnose this condition, but a D & C is more accurate because all the endometrium is removed.

The two main types of endometrial hyperplasia are cystic and adenomatous. Cystic is an over-growth of *normal* cells and can often be reversed with medication. Adenomatous, especially where the pathology report says 'atypical cells' or 'atypical hyperplasia', is akin to carcinoma in situ (CIS) and is more closely associated with development into cancer. In young women hormones are often given as treatment and there can be a spontaneous cure as they grow older. Older women are less likely to have a spontaneous cure, so a D & C as diagnosis is more important. There is a continuum of hyperplastic changes in the endometrium, and it is important to have a clear understanding of which diagnosis you have.

It is important to find out what your histology report says; you are quite entitled to have a copy of it. The histologic diagnosis from the D & C will influence the treatment. If it is cystic, a further D & C and treatment with progesterone might be suggested; if adenomatous, a hysterectomy with possible removal of tubes and ovaries as well would probably be recommended. A young woman who has adenomatous hyperplasia but who wishes to have children may decide to have hormones and a repeat D & C. She should be aware of the risk she is taking and be prepared to commit herself to careful follow-up with repeat endometrial biopsies.

Uterine cancer

Cancer of the corpus (body) of the uterus (as opposed to the cervix) can be endometrial (of the lining) or a sarcoma (highly malignant tumour) of the connective or muscle tissue of the uterus. The latter is extremely rare and is often not detected until it is well advanced. The treatment is radical hysterectomy, radiation or chemotherapy.

Endometrial cancer is uncommon, but seems to be increasing. It is mostly found in women aged 55–74 (it causes 6 percent of cancers in this age group). The cause is unknown, but is thought to be linked to the hormone oestrogen. Women who have high levels of oestrogen are at risk. These are very overweight women who have excess oestrogen in their fatty tissue, childless women, women who have a late menopause and who therefore have more years of oestrogen stimulation, and women on oestrogen replacement therapy.

Abnormal bleeding is the most common symptom of endometrial cancer. In pre-menopausal women prolonged periods, a sudden flow, or staining between periods or after intercourse can be a sign. In post-menopausal women skipping periods, tapering off, spotting or stopping and starting can all be signs. The causes of any of this bleeding in pre- or post-menopausal women can be quite harmless, but about a third of abnormal bleeding in post-menopausal women will be caused by endometrial or cervical cancer. Any type of bleeding after menopause should be carefully investigated.

Vaginal discharge or a sudden burst of watery fluid after exertion or straining on the lavatory can be symptoms. A brown or blood-tinged smelly discharge may mean a pyometra, a build-up of blood or pus in the uterus.

An endometrial biopsy might diagnose endometrial cancer but a D & C is more accurate. During the procedure the uterus is measured because a larger uterus can indicate a later stage of the disease. In stages I and II of endometrial cancer the cancer is confined to the body of the uterus; in stages III and IV, the cancer has spread to adjacent tissue and then to other organs.

Endometrial cancer nearly always involves the removal of the uterus and vaginal cuff, the upper part of the vagina. The tubes and ovaries may be removed and if the disease has spread, the lymph nodes. In a very few cases pelvic exenteration is performed, removing the vagina, rectum and bladder. This is very extensive surgery with a poor outcome and it is very rarely resorted to.

Radiation therapy by radioactive implants or external radiation is frequently given before surgery. This alters the cancer cells, making it impossible for them to implant elsewhere, and scars the blood vessels and lymph nodes in the area so that the chances of spreading the cancer cells during surgery are reduced. These therapies are the same as those for cervical cancer.

If a woman is obese, there are sometimes limits to the extent of surgery that can safely be undertaken. A prolonged anaesthetic could pose quite a risk. There are many variations in treatment given and this is decided according to the extent of the disease and the woman's general health. Women need to be given a full description of the treatments offered and their short-term and long-term effects when deciding what treatment to undergo.

Cervical carcinoma in situ
Carcinoma in situ is an abnormal condition of the cells in the epithelium (surface skin) of the cervix. If it is not treated it can develop into invasive cervical cancer, where the deeper layers of cells are affected. The disease can then spread to other parts of the body. Because CIS is not invasive, some doctors call it a cancer precursor, or pre-cancer.

CIS also has a number of other names, including severe

dysplasia and CIN 3. CIN stands for cervical intraepithelial neoplasia, which means new growth within the epithelium. CIN is graded 1, 2 or 3, with 3 being the most severe condition.

CIS has no symptoms and it is usually detected by a cervical smear test. Before any treatment is undertaken, it is essential that an accurate diagnosis is made and a smear test cannot do this by itself. A smear test might under-report or over-report, that is, suggest something less or more than is actually there.

The next step should always be colposcopy, which magnifies the cervix and shows up abnormalities; the doctor will also take a small biopsy. The tissue is sent to a laboratory for an accurate diagnosis. If it shows CIS, the treatment will be discussed with the patient.

The aim of treatment is to remove all the diseased cells. Twenty years ago, hysterectomy was almost always used; today more limited methods of treatment are usually used, especially if the woman wants children. The following methods are called locally destructive treatments:

- Diathermy burns the cells away.
- Cryocautery or cryosurgery freezes the cells.
- Laser vaporises the cells. Laser is a new treatment only available in the biggest public hospitals or in some private clinics.

The advantage of these treatments is that they damage the cervix as little as possible, which will be important if you want to have more children, and they can be done under a local anaesthetic without the need for a stay in hospital.

In another treatment, called cone biopsy, a cone-shaped piece of tissue is cut from the cervix to take away all the abnormal cells. A cone biopsy involves a day or two in hospital, and there are risks (such as haemorrhage, or a less functional cervix), but it is a very effective means of treating CIS.

After a cone biopsy you can ask to see the laboratory report. If the lab reports 'incomplete excision margins' or indicates in some way that not all the abnormal cells have been removed, you should consider more extensive treatment. Occasionally, in the healing process after a cone biopsy, any remaining abnormal cells will be destroyed, so that further treatment might not be needed.

A method used to treat CIS in some hospitals is Cartier excision, which uses an electric wire to slice away the abnormal tissue. It is a less extensive treatment than cone biopsy, but the tissue removed can still be sent to the laboratory for a report. In the locally destructive methods, tissue is not available for the histologists, and it is follow-up reports which show if the treatment has been successful. A recent extension of Cartier excision is called a Leitz biopsy. In this method the abnormal tissue is cut out with a large metal loop.

A woman with CIS might consider a hysterectomy if:

- She has completed her family
- She has had one or two local treatments and still has abnormal smears or colposcopy
- A cone biopsy has not removed all the abnormal tissue
- She has other problems with her uterus, for example, fibroids or heavy, painful periods
- She wants a method of permanent sterilisation.

The advantage of hysterectomy is that it is more likely to remove all the abnormal tissue. It is still necessary to have follow-up smears of the vaginal vault although it does not need to be as frequent as if one of the other methods had been used. Some women may find the close follow-up after a local method irksome and worrying. Of course, a woman who chooses a hysterectomy will have to consider the fact that it is major surgery and that there are possible complications.

There are great variations in medical opinion about the best treatment for women with CIS. For example, some doctors will recommend hysterectomy for CIS as the first option. Others suggest a third locally destructive treatment when two previous attempts have been unsuccessful. This can make it very hard for you to be sure of the best course of action. Your own doctor may recommend a treatment while another may advise something different. It is a good idea to get a second opinion if you are doubtful about what is suggested to you and, in the end, it is your decision. You are the one who has to live with the outcome of the decision, so it is important that you feel happy about it. For further information on the disease and its treatments, read *Cervical Cancer* by Linda Dyson (see Bibliography).

Microinvasive cervical cancer

The first stage of invasion is called microinvasive cancer or Stage Ia cervical cancer. The disease has invaded only about 3–5mm. Because the cancer is confined, the doctor might suggest a simple cone biopsy if you wish to have children, with very close follow-up, and possibly a hysterectomy later. Otherwise, a simple hysterectomy with close follow-up would probably be considered adequate treatment. It is important you feel able to discuss fully the implications of the diagnosis and treatment with your doctor. Although CIS does not always progress to invasion, with microinvasion the process has already begun.

Invasive cervical cancer

It was extremely perturbing that a few women completing the hysterectomy questionnaire gave as their reason for having a hysterectomy 'suspected' or 'possible' cancer. One woman said she had a hysterectomy for 'a lump thought to be cancer'. Another said, 'I was advised to have it as cancer is in the family.' There is no evidence that cervical cancer runs in families. Doctors should always know for certain whether there is cancer before they start treatment. Treating the wrong thing can have disastrous consequences if there is undertreatment or if the treatment is more radical than is necessary. It is quite possible to make that diagnosis accurately, so women should, if necessary, insist on having a diagnosis written down and explained.

Cervical cancer is not very common, although the great

increase in cancer precursors has led some doctors to talk of an epidemic in younger women. Each year about 200 women have invasive cervical cancer diagnosed, and 100 will die of it. It is the second most frequent cancer in the 15–34 age group (melanoma 29 percent, cervix 16 percent) and the fourth most frequent in the 35–54 age group (8 percent, after breast, bowel and melanoma). It causes 17 percent of cancer deaths in women aged 15–34, and 7 percent in the 35–54 age group.

Unlike CIS, invasive cancer can have symptoms. You should consult your doctor if you notice:

- Changes in menstruation especially a heavier, longer flow
- A brown or bloody discharge
- Bleeding after intercourse
- Bleeding between periods or after menopause
- Low back and sciatic nerve pain.

These can all be symptoms of other, benign disorders, but should be carefully checked out. The cervix can still look normal to the naked eye, although sometimes there is visible abnormality, such as an ulcer, and the cervix might bleed when touched.

Colposcopy and biopsy would be carried out, although if the doctor is very suspicious she or he might suggest a bigger biopsy under anaesthetic at which time a thorough vaginal and rectal examination would be carried out. Sometimes the cancer can be felt as a hard area, and at this point the doctors would 'stage' the disease.

All cancers are staged according to the extent of the spread of the disease. Stage 1a, 1b and even 2a cervical cancers have a good chance of being successfully treated. The survival rate for 1a and 1b after five years is 86 percent. The survival rates of stage 2a and 2b cancers is 54 percent; those for 3 and 4 cancers are not as good. Generally cervical cancer is one of the most successfully treated cancers because the uterus is accessible and not necessary for survival, unlike, for example, the liver.

Treatment for invasive cancer involves a radical kind of

hysterectomy, called a Wertheim's hysterectomy. This involves the removal of uterus, tubes and ovaries as well as the lymph nodes and tissue adjacent to the uterus. Before the surgery the malignant cells are destroyed by radiation therapy.

For later stage cancer, surgery may not be performed because the disease has spread too far to be contained by surgery. The treatment would usually consist of a course of external radiation, beamed through the pelvis from the outside and, following that, insertion of radioactive caesium rods in the cervical canal.

Ovarian cancer

Ovarian cancer accounts for 5 percent of cancers and 9 percent of female cancer deaths in the 35–54 age group, but is most common in women over 50. In all age groups, ovarian cancer accounts for 4 percent of female cancer deaths, reflecting the fact that while it is less common than cervical cancer, it does not have such a good cure rate, as it is difficult to detect and therefore is often not discovered until it is at an advanced stage.

A woman who has never had children is 2.5 times more likely to develop ovarian cancer than one who has been pregnant 3 or more times. There may be a family history of ovarian cancer, and prior breast, endometrial or colon cancer increases the chance of developing ovarian cancer.

Malignant growths in the ovaries appear as cysts or tumours and are usually detected because the woman or her doctor feels a lump on one or both sides of her abdomen. Cysts can also cause pain, an enlarged abdomen, menstrual disturbances, constipation and a general feeling of being unwell, with nausea and weight loss. Cysts can also be benign, so it is not until it is removed or sampled and a pathology report is made that malignancy can be ruled out or confirmed. In younger women tumours are more likely to be benign; in post-menopausal women, 50 percent of tumours are cancerous.

Ovarian cancer is staged in a similar way to cervical cancer and endometrial cancer and the treatment involves surgery, often followed by some form of chemotherapy. Even early stage ovarian cancer involves the removal of the tubes and uterus as well as the ovaries, unless the woman is young, when only the ovaries might be removed. In very early stage cancer, chemotherapy might be omitted. At the time of the surgery, cells should be collected from the area. If these are positive for cancer, chemotherapy would be recommended but if they are negative, chemotherapy would probably be omitted on the assumption that the surgery has contained the disease.

Careful follow-up and checks are important for women who have been treated for ovarian cancer. Good nutrition is important after ovarian cancer and as women who have had ovarian cancer are at higher risk of breast cancer, regular breast checks are necessary. The five-year survival rate for ovarian cancer is 30 percent overall, although there is a great difference in rates according to the type of tumour. Some stage 1 tumours have a better than 95 percent survival rate.

6

MAKING THE DECISION

What women in our survey knew

Our questionnaire results revealed that the majority of the women were hardly informed at all of the risks of hysterectomy, or even what to expect during the recovery time.

Thirty-two percent of women completing the questionnaire said they did not feel they were given enough information by their doctors to give informed consent. But even though two-thirds of the women felt they had been given enough information to make the decision, only a minority of these were actually warned of negative effects. When asked if they had been told of any possible negative effects of hysterectomy, 68 percent of the women said 'no', while only 32 percent ticked 'yes'.

Depression was the negative effect doctors most frequently told women about: 18 percent of the women had been told this might happen. Around 15 percent of women were warned about hot flushes, 12 percent of mood changes and 11 percent of bowel and bladder problems. Seven percent were told about the possibility of haemorrhage or infection. Three percent were told about the chance of a less satisfactory sex life and about the same percentage that they could have difficulty reaching orgasm.

There was no correlation between being informed about a possible negative effect and actually experiencing it, which contradicts the old medical myth that if you tell women about possible complications, they'll get them.

61

A good number of women filling out the questionnaire commented that they had found the article accompanying it extremely helpful. It mentioned feelings and complications that they had had, but had no idea were experienced by other women. One woman said that reading that scar tissue at the top of the vagina could occasionally cause pain if it was aggravated during intercourse provided her with an explanation for the discomfort she had been experiencing for 15 years. Another woman said she felt so relieved to have her own experience validated, she burst into tears while reading the article. 'I actually cried when reading your article as I had thought that perhaps I was the only one to have difficulties adjusting.'

Three percent of the women did not know what organs had been removed and a further 2 percent were uncertain. One who had her operation in 1976 wrote: 'Still don't know. Doctor said ovaries could go, when I asked, was told "Not to worry".' Another said:

All the surgeon told me was that I should have an abdominal hysterectomy because I had fibroids which could become cancerous. He did not explain anything about the operation at all . . . Before I left the hospital, I asked the surgeon what he had removed and what I could do or not do and all he said was 'Don't go moving any pianos, ha ha!'

Another woman wrote:

I read your article four days after I had a hysterectomy, and it told me more about the operation than my doctor had told me . . . I was reading it when the nurse came around. I tried to speak to her about it, but was told, if you want to believe everything you read that's up to you.

This woman had gone under the anaesthetic believing she had cancer. Three months earlier she had had a grade 3 cervical smear. Three days after the operation, the doctor told her she had only had an infection. Her experience, in 1987, highlights the abysmal lack of knowledge suffered by some women both before and after the operation.

Why women should be fully informed

Making such an important decision as whether to have a hysterectomy requires that we have all the information so that we can make an informed choice. There is research to confirm the view that people cope better with hysterectomy when they are well informed. Many women in our survey expressed similar feelings to this: 'I would like to see doctors giving adequate counselling to patients about to undergo hysterectomy. I think I would have coped a lot better if I had been told of possible negative aspects after the operation. I was informed of all the positive things about it.'

Even when women asked questions, they did not always get answers. One woman wrote: 'I asked questions but was treated as though I was looking for problems in a routine and simple procedure. I was not prepared in any way for the complications that followed.'

It has been argued that fully informing women would 'put them off having necessary surgery'. We contend that if women are 'put off' by the facts, that is their right. But we doubt that droves of women would be 'put off' by the truth; they would simply cope better.

Because doctors had not always given women enough information, some had done their own homework. They had read books from shops or the library and had asked other women.

Some doctors had taken time to inform their patients and there was even one who had prepared his own leaflet, although the tone of it was very patronising. A few doctors provided leaflets of varying quality or lent books, including the excellent manual by Lorraine Dennerstein, Carl Wood and Graham Burrows. These doctors were in the minority. Some doctors included women's partners in their consultation and this was appreciated.

Given that this is a very commonly performed operation, we feel it is surprising and remiss that doctors' professional bodies have failed to provide information in a systematic way. The American College of Obstetricians and Gynaecologists, for example, has produced a pamphlet on hysterectomy for women as part of a patient education scheme. Similar projects would be welcome in New Zealand.

One of our respondents described a hospital where great care was taken to prepare women.

> I was given a folder on hysterectomy prepared by a sister who had had the operation. It stated clearly versions of technique, how it was done, e.g. external, internal, how they cut, etc. How you were prepared. What to expect on arrival back from theatre and in the days to come. Stitches, drips, drains, etc. Things to do and not to do. Sexual, etc. This I found beaut. They also asked husbands to read, which he did and then a nurse came and discussed how we felt. I would have been asked by a least four different nurses did I know all I wanted to. To us it was all very clear and totally acceptable . . . Now seven years on, I can do everything I did in my early twenties. We were warned it would affect our sex life, but after an initial decline, it's as good as ever. The quality of my life is 300% better.

Unlike this woman, an alarming number of women had entered hospital in ignorance about their situation. Some then had feelings of shock, anger and bitterness when they experienced problems, or even normal repercussions of having a hysterectomy. One wrote: 'I wasn't prepared for waking up to find an IV in my arm or drainage tubes hanging on both sides of the bed. This was a shock.' Another woman wrote: 'It was only after the operation that I received an awful shock when using the commode provided to find that I was bleeding. The sister explained, but I did feel a fool and wished I had been previously prepared for this.'

Another was well prepared for the operation, but not for possible complications. 'The surgeon I saw was great, taking the time to explain. He was very gentle.' This woman wanted to see the womb: 'It was shown to me as soon as it was removed. I was amazed at how small it was! How could that little thing cause so much pain! . . . But I don't remember being told of any negative side-effects either by my own doctor or the surgeon.' She had sustained bladder damage during the operation and despite a further operation still leaks urine. In general she feels positive about the operation, but 'my bladder seems to be worse than ever, I'm always wanting to go to the toilet, which makes me very angry'.

Some were stunned to find they felt so ill and helpless afterwards; they had not expected it and found it difficult to cope with. Others experienced effects that some doctors deny are possible. Most of the existing leaflets on hysterectomy state categorically that there will be no difference in sexual enjoyment, that there may be a short-term emotional reaction, and that hot flushes will only occur if the ovaries are removed. Our survey of women confirmed what some overseas writers have observed, that this is an inaccurate underplaying of the possible effects of hysterectomy. A significant number of women commented that they would not have gone ahead with the operation had they known 'what I know now'.

One woman (aged 43) wrote:

> The mood swings I was not prepared for. I go from grim determination with a 'stuff the lot of them' attitude, to tears of frustration. I don't think I have ever cried so much in my life. By profession I am a high school teacher. I say this because I am normally in control of things and having the hysterectomy has made my life fall apart. I don't think had I been given any literature I would have agreed to it.

Another, aged 31, who like the above woman had only her womb removed, also had swinging moods.

> It was so bad between my husband and I that we split, spending 11 months apart before we finally decided to have another go at

our marriage. I did ask my own GP if I should be experiencing mood changes and he told me not to be so silly. I knew at the time there was nothing else to be done except have the hysterectomy, but would have liked to know what to expect afterwards. I feel better to know that others have felt like I did and it wasn't just me.

A 46-year-old woman who had her hysterectomy in 1976 wrote:

Internal pleasure has seriously deteriorated and intercourse has never since produced orgasm. Had I been warned this was possible, I'd have tried to avoid hysterectomy and opted for a bladder repair. The surgeon was a kindly enough man, but I felt passed onto him like a factory product such was the 'routine, no argument, no discussion, nothing to it' attitude of my GP in those days. I gather now that there was much more to the op than I was told.

How well do hospitals inform women?

In preparing this book, we wrote to all public hospitals in New Zealand performing hysterectomies as well as a selection of private hospitals. We asked how many hysterectomies they performed and for what reasons. We also asked what counselling and support they could provide for women, and for copies of any informational material they made available to women.

Unfortunately, while the smaller public hospitals provided statistical material, the larger hospitals and private hospitals did not. It was not possible either to obtain this information from the Government, as some hospital superintendents suggested. Under the Government's user-pays policy, we were to be charged and our budget did not allow it.

However, most of the hospitals did respond to the questions about support and informational material. Several of the hospitals sent copies of *Curing the Hysterectomy Hang-ups*, an outdated leaflet produced in the early 1970s and much criticised by women's groups. Occasionally a hospital had gone to quite a lot of trouble to produce a leaflet for patients, although these were of varying quality.

None of the leaflets covered indications for hysterectomy, the expectation being that the decision for hysterectomy had already been taken. The emphasis tended to be on how quickly the woman could resume her household tasks, for example, lifting washing, vacuuming and ironing. The risks were generally underplayed and major long-term risks, such as bladder damage, not mentioned at all. One hospital offered the Dennerstein book, which is realistic about after-effects. All the other informational material we were sent stated baldly that women could expect to be unchanged by hysterectomy, to have a short weepy period followed by a speedy return to a normal emotional state, no detrimental sexual repercussions, and that only if the ovaries were removed could menopausal symptoms be expected.

Palmerston North was the only hospital that offered a hysterectomy support group, run by women who had already had the operation. In most hospitals, the surgeon or nurses were deemed adequate to provide counselling. There was no organised ongoing support such as is available in some places for women having abortions, colposcopy, repeated miscarriages or in infertility programmes. This may reflect medical attitudes that hysterectomy is no big deal and thus should receive no 'special' support services. Some hospitals pointed out that hospital social workers were available, although it was not clear how women would know about this.

One women vividly expressed her need for support. She was 41 when she had the operation in 1968.

I needed to talk to someone but could not initiate this myself. Hysterectomy was regarded as commonplace and routine, which in one sense was true. To a single or childless woman it was far from so and brought a strong sense of aloneness, deprivation and desolation. The approach to talking about it would have to have come from outside and by offer, as I was unable then to verbalise feelings or to approach anyone.

Another woman described how important the help of the hospital physiotherapist had been.

> We were given excellent information and encouragement the evening before our operations . . . she gave us confidence, encouragement and a positive outlook, and all the necessary tips to cope with convalescing. She told us exactly what to expect at hospital and at home. Maybe she was exceptional; I was most grateful to her. It was not until I was in hospital that I found out I would not be able to do anything much for six weeks — just as well my children were teenagers.

Despite the prevalence of hysterectomy, little has been done within the health system to assist women in deciding about it, and coping with it at the time or afterwards.

Talking to your doctor about hysterectomy

You will want to ask your doctor many questions about your condition and the likelihood hysterectomy will cure it. As a broad guideline, the questions you might want to ask could be:

- What condition do I have?
- What has caused my condition?
- What will happen if it is not treated?
- What alternative treatments are there and what are the chances they would be successful?
- What parts of my body will be removed?
- What likelihood is there of hysterectomy curing or improving my condition.
- Which symptoms will be cured, and which will not?
- Is my condition cancerous or malignant? (Make sure the doctor distinguishes clearly between malignancy and a pre-cancerous condition.)
- What risks am I taking?
- What effects of the surgery can I expect?
- What benefits can I expect?

Ask for diagrams to be drawn, for language you can understand to be used, and for terms that are new to be written down. Get a diagnosis in writing. Ask for copies of laboratory reports, especially if cancer or a pre-cancer is involved.

In public hospitals, you have a legal right to look at your records. The situation in a private hospital is not so clear. The New Zealand Medical Association has made a ruling that doctors should share their files with patients, and that any diagnoses and laboratory or pathology reports belong to the patient. However, not all doctors belong to the Medical Association and practices vary widely.

It is necessary for us to state that you have an absolute right to refuse a hysterectomy. Some women who answered our questionnaire felt that this was a decision for the doctor, and not them. One wrote: 'I did not know I could have refused. I was told I didn't need my womb any more.'

When faced with a strong opinion from an obviously knowledgeable authority figure, such as a medical specialist, some women feel quite overawed and unassertive. But it is you who are having the operation, it is your body, your feelings, and you can say no or that you want time to consider it.

A critical part of decision-making is knowledge about the risks you are taking. Some doctors think it is better to 'protect' patients from the 'bad news', so as not to worry them unnecessarily. This paternalistic, old-fashioned attitude is no longer acceptable, if it ever was. It implies that women are not adult and mature enough to make sensible decisions, to take in negative as well as positive information and balance risks and benefits. It perpetuates the idea that the doctor knows best. By withholding information, the doctor is actually denying patients control over their own bodies. When things go wrong, the patient feels betrayed and loses trust.

Second opinions and changing your doctor

If you would like to have an opinion from another doctor about your condition, you have a right to this. It is commonplace in some other countries, but occasionally a New Zealand doctor will be affronted. In public hospitals another hospital doctor could do this, although you may wonder how independent that opinion will be. It is preferable the doctor is in another team from the first one. To find a doctor for a second opinion in the private sector, ask your specialist, GP, family planning clinic or women's health centre, or canvass friends.

If you encounter difficulty with your doctor over any of these matters you should consider whether that doctor is an appropriate adviser for you. This can be a hard decision, as it is possible that a doctor who is not so good at communicating is the best available surgeon. Changing your doctor might also not be easy if you live in a small town or have a complaint where a specialised opinion might be necessary. It may be necessary to travel to a larger centre to find an appropriate gynaecologist.

Taking your partner or a friend with you when you visit the specialist can be a help. That person can also make sure you ask all the questions in your mind — discuss them together and write them down beforehand. He or she can also help make sure you get answers, and help with remembering what you were told afterwards. It is advisable to inform a doctor you will have someone with you when making an appointment, but it is your right to have your own personal friend and advocate with you.

Don't be hurried

Give yourself time to consider your feelings, and discuss the matter with family and friends. You might decide to give some alternative therapies, such as herbal treatments or acupuncture, a try first.

Beware of the doctor in the private sector who wants to book you in to a private hospital very quickly. Cancers must be treated urgently, but this will almost certainly be in a public hospital, which will have the specialised equipment to perform this surgery. For other cases there is usually no great urgency. If a private specialist says you should go into a private hospital because there is a lengthy waiting list to get into a public hospital, check yourself, or ask your GP to check. We do know of cases where waiting times have been exaggerated by specialists.

Professor Hutton reported that in his experience cancer patients are among the people who adjust worst to hysterectomy, not just because they have a life-threatening condition, but because they have no choice, and because they have no time to get used to the idea. There are benefits, he believes, in waiting lists.

Questions you might have in your mind while making a decision are:

- How much is my condition affecting the quality of my life and my plans for the future? What is it stopping me doing?
- How does it affect other important people in my life?
- How do I feel about the loss of my uterus and about not menstruating? What do they mean to me?
- Is my family completed? Do I want more children?
- What will happen if I don't have a hysterectomy?
- What does my husband or sexual partner think about it?
- Are there things I or other people can do to make it a comfortable decision?

You might consider penning 'After hysterectomy' and 'Not having a hysterectomy' scenarios and looking at which you would rather be in!

7

HOW WOMEN FEEL ABOUT HYSTERECTOMY

Hysterectomy is not just an operation. It has a special significance for many women. One of the reasons hysterectomy may be recommended too lightly is that doctors don't always understand these feelings. They think that women will be glad to get rid of periods and that the uterus is redundant once a woman has completed her family.

There were women who answered our questionnaire who said that losing their uterus was no big deal.

> In fact, if I had to lose anything, apart from my appendix, that appeared to be the most dispensable.

> There is a mild regret that I had to lose part of my body, but I regret much more losing two front teeth when I was twelve years old, and having to wear a partial plate since then.

Many women, however, value their wombs very highly. They feel the womb has significance over and above its actual reproductive function and may feel that their sense of bodily intactness, their completeness as a woman and their sexual desirability are closely associated with it.

This woman was advised to have a hysterectomy for heavy bleeding when she was 35 years old, even though she would have liked another child. She had many reactions.

I felt as though I had lost not only my womb, my sexuality and potential to be a mother again but also that child I was looking forward to having. But I kept being told I was lucky to have two lovely children and no more periods. But I felt good about having periods. It was like the rhythm of the seasons. I was always regular and when it came it felt like 'all's right with the world'.

I worried about lots of little things, like what happens to the egg each month, and what happens to the semen during intercourse. And what would I look like inside now, because I had to change the body image of myself.

Many women who answered our questionnaire talked about being sad about not being able to have more children. Thirteen percent of the women said they felt grief at their loss of fertility. Younger women who had not had children could feel devastated.

I felt shattered emotionally when told I was to have a hysterectomy. I bargained a lot with myself, God and doctors — anything but not being able to have kids. I felt guilty about a past abortion, and felt that hysterectomy was my punishment. I felt inadequate as a woman — what did I have to offer a relationship?

But even women who had decided to have no children or no more children could find what one woman called 'the terrible finality' was difficult to face. Women's reactions to hysterectomy can be very complex and not at all predictable.

I can remember having a cry before the operation for the fact that I would not be able to have more children — this may seem silly as I was 35, had three lovely girls and [we] had no intention of having more children. It was just that I knew that this was *it* and I loved my babies. These feelings however did not override my feelings of relief — also my husband was a great help emotionally.

I thought a hysterectomy would be no hassle for me, a nun, because of the choice I made 23 years ago to live a life of celibate love. But there were some very serious things I needed to think about before saying yes to surgery. One of these was the possibility of having 'taken back', or no longer having 'the gift of celibacy' in relation to God, because of the removal of the womb. Another was the realisation that the physical possibility of motherhood would no longer be there — this still had to be taken hold of and internalised, despite my choice of lifestyle . . . I became acutely aware of my own femininity, and the realisation that my uterus was in a very real sense my 'heart'. My sexuality is the source of my energy to love, and to receive love, and it is a very integral part of my being. I had to be assured, and believe, that this part of me would not be impaired or destroyed through hysterectomy. I received this assurance.

It was often very difficult to come to the decision, even if there were clear indications it should be done: 'Surgery brought about a dichotomy between what I knew, and what I felt. I knew it was necessary, but I was unreconciled to it. I accepted rationally that it needed to be done, but not emotionally — so hard to say "yes" when all your emotions are screaming "no".'

In our questionnaire we asked women to describe in their own words their feelings at the time of the hysterectomy. Forty-three percent described only positive feelings about the hysterectomy; 35 percent negative ones; and 18 percent had both positive and negative feelings, or mixed feelings; 6 percent were neutral or uncertain about their feelings.

Some of the positive words people used were 'hopeful', 'decided', 'determined', 'excited', 'confident', and 'relieved'.

When I was told I could have a hysterectomy I was over the moon! After years of very heavy bleeding, terrible pain, cramps, PMT, etc, not to mention pain during and after intercourse, I was delighted to see an end to it all.

I was fortunate to have two lovely children so having a hysterectomy was a positive step. Back to health.

I knew it was very necessary as I ended up going into hospital with each period to get pain relief that worked. I was quite happy to have it done as I had a week to ten days being very sick with my period and another three to four days at ovulation. I had become a burden to my family because of this.

The people who felt negative used words like 'trapped', 'anxious', 'terrified', 'stunned', 'bewildered', 'numb', 'tense', and 'uncertain.'

Sometimes women felt that by not having to wait too long before surgery, they had avoided mounting panic, but others felt very hassled at having insufficient time: 'I felt I was on a roller coaster — ups and downs and it's all happening too fast, and I couldn't stop to think it all out.'

In answer to this part of the questionnaire about their feelings at the time of their hysterectomy women could write about anything they liked. The majority of the feelings women expressed were about the operation ahead, what they had to go through and their reaction to it. Many of these feelings related to not knowing exactly what was going on and what to expect. Eleven percent of our respondents also said they felt negative about aspects of the health care system. They mentioned 'bungled' health care, 'arrogant' and 'abrupt' doctors, being intimidated and not having enough information given to them. Previous negative experiences with health professionals didn't help these women face their upcoming operation in a very good frame of mind.

> I welcomed the operation as I was told I would feel a 'new woman' — but little else. I didn't know till I was admitted to hospital that I would have a vaginal hysterectomy and repair. The doctor was abrupt and I was left bewildered but being a quiet person accepted my fate.

Women mentioned being nervous about the anaesthetic, loss of privacy, and about pain. Frequently the fear of the unknown added to their anxiety.

> Fear of the unknown is horrid and frightening. No matter how much the (men) specialists said 'don't worry' and my boyfriend was loving, I still had that huge question mark — how will I be? What will it feel like? The fear was heightened also because I had

never been to hospital and had not been to doctors (I don't suffer sickness usually).

Being unwell added to negative feelings before the operation. Some of the women were simply too sick and exhausted to cope well. Fifteen percent of the women mentioned this feeling, using words like 'worn out', 'drained', 'sore', 'rotten', and 'debilitated'.

They also worried about how their families would cope while they were in hospital, especially if they had young children, or how long it would be before they got back to their jobs. Women wanted to organise their families before going into hospital so they could cope in their absence, and be ready to care for them when they came home.

It would be abnormal not to have anxieties before major surgery, but for the majority of the women who answered our questionnaire, however, the idea of going into hospital was a manageable stress.

Maori women

As we noted in Chapter One, few Maori women responded to our questionnaire, and those who did made no comments about their race, apart from one respondent who felt that Maori women were expected to put up with more pain after the operation than Pakeha women. Because of this low response rate, we know little about the way Maori women might respond differently to hysterectomy. Professor Mantell, who is himself Maori, had, he said, experienced no difference in Maori women's attitudes.

In some overseas countries, race has an influence on hysterectomy rates. In America, there is concern about hysterectomy rates for black women and the effect on their sexuality. Fears have been expressed that unnecessary hysterectomies have been performed on black women to reduce the black population. New York State Department of Health statistics show that in New York State, for example, hysterectomy rates in 1988 for black women aged 30 to 59 were nearly 50 percent higher than those for white women.

This pattern does not appear to be repeated in New Zealand. Health Department statistics show that Maori women are actually less likely to have hysterectomies. For women over 20, the rate is around 6 per 1 000 women for Pakeha women, and 4 per 1 000 for Maori women.

Traditionally, Maori people have strong beliefs about both the female reproductive organs and the loss of body parts. At the Commission of Inquiry into the Treatment of Cervical Cancer at National Women's Hospital, Te Ohu Whakatupu, the Maori unit of the Ministry of Women's Affairs, gave submissions on Maori aspects of the inquiry. They stated that: 'Te whare o te tangata [the house of the people], the reproductive system of women is in Maori terms highly valued as the procreative home of humankind. It provides the sheltering environment for all generations. It contributes to mana wahine [the status of women] . . . te whare o te tangata is a taonga, a treasure to be protected.'

Te Ohu also pointed out that the links between the female reproductive system and the tribe and family were so strong that 'terms that describe different social groups also mean different stages of reproduction. Whanau not only means the extended family but also means birth and the birth process.'

'The term hapu refers not only to the tribe or subtribe but also means to be pregnant. The link between the woman and nurturing and sustenance of the people is also made with the common definition of whenua. Not only does whenua mean the land but it also means the placenta . . .'

The Maori people had developed many rituals around menstruation and birth, some of which, such as taking the placenta back to bury on the family land, are still followed by some Maori people today. In addition, blood and body parts, even hair and nail clippings, are still considered to be part of the body, even when removed from it. Such things would be handled and disposed of very carefully, because someone with evil intent could harm the person through the body parts.

Even when removed, said Te Ohu Whakatupu, 'the uterus still is a part of that person, it has a life-force of its own.' While they explained that modern Maori women did not all think this way, many still held to some of these traditional beliefs and practices.

How widespread these attitudes are, and how they affect Maori women's response to hysterectomy, we do not know, but for Maori women there may be additional factors in their decision-making, and different adjustments to make.

8

HOW THE OPERATION
IS DONE

Types of hysterectomy operation

There are several different types of hysterectomy and you should
be clear about exactly what is proposed for you.

Sub-total hysterectomy
This removes the body or fundus of the uterus but not the cervix.
It is not often performed today, as the cervix is almost always
removed too. Hospital figures for 1985 show that only 52 out of
over 6 000 hysterectomies performed in 1985 were sub-total. The
arguments for removing the cervix are that it has no function
without the uterus, and it could become cancerous. These reasons
are not very convincing and a re-evaluation of routine removal of
the cervix is needed. Of course, the cervix can be a potential site
for disease, but organs shouldn't be removed on the basis that
they *might* become diseased in the future.

If a woman has had abnormal smears, such as carcinoma in situ,
she might be relieved to have her cervix removed when she has a
hysterectomy, as she has a greater (though still slim) chance of
developing cancer. But in many cases the cervices being removed
are, and always have been, perfectly healthy.

By retaining the cervix, the chance of women experiencing less
satisfactory sex after hysterectomy may be lessened. The top of

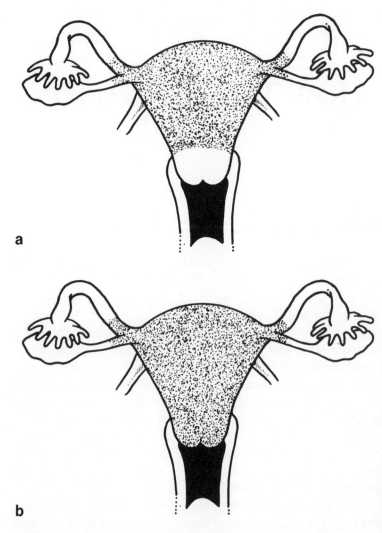

Different types of hysterectomy. The shaded area shows tissue which is removed.

a. *Sub-total hysterectomy. The cervix remains.*
b. *Total or simple hysterectomy. The uterus and cervix are removed (and sometimes the Fallopian tubes as well).*

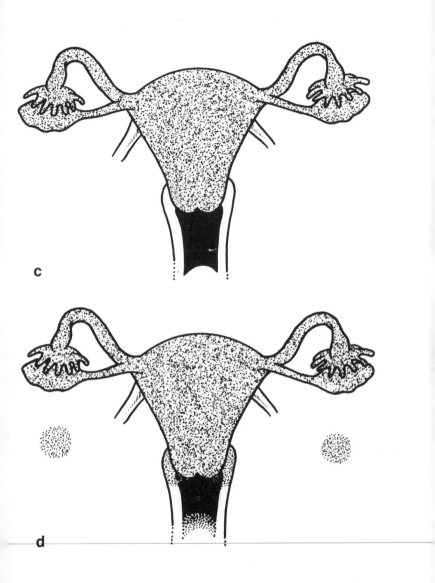

c. *Total hysterectomy plus bilateral salpingo-oophorectomy. Uterus, cervix, both tubes and ovaries are removed.*

d. *Radical or Wertheim's hysterectomy. The uterus, cervix, tubes, ovaries, upper vagina and pelvic lymph nodes are removed.*

the vagina would be unaltered and the part the cervix and vaginal vault play in sexual excitement might not be affected. Research on this topic would be valuable.

A statistical survey of hysterectomies in New York state found that the mortality for sub-total operations is higher than that for total ones.

Total or simple hysterectomy
This is the most commonly performed operation. The fundus and cervix are removed. After removal of the uterus, the top of the vagina is sewn up so that it is closed off at the top. The other organs rearrange themselves to take up the small space formerly occupied by the uterus. The eggs released by the ovaries each month are simply absorbed into the body as they also are after tubal ligation. During abdominal surgery the Fallopian tubes are often removed, especially if there is some disease such as endometriosis or pelvic inflammatory disease. This is something you should discuss with your doctor beforehand as part of being clear about what organs are being removed.

Total hysterectomy plus bilateral salpingo-oophorectomy
The whole uterus is removed as well as the Fallopian tubes (salpingo-) and ovaries (oophorectomy).

Radical hysterectomy or Wertheim's hysterectomy
Used only for cancer treatment, this operation usually involves irradiation of the pelvis using radioactive rods to sterilise the cancer cells, followed by surgical removal of the uterus and adjacent tissue, such as the pelvic lymph nodes, the parametrial tissue and the vaginal cuff at the top of the vagina. The amount removed will vary according to the spread of the cancer and should be fully explained by the surgeon

The radioactive rods or the casing to hold them are fitted in the operating theatre. On returning to the ward the woman has to lie flat for 24–36 hours behind lead shields. Visitors are kept to a minimum. She can then go home, returning about four weeks later for surgery. If the cancer has spread, post-surgery radiotherapy may be carried out. There is a very full description of these treatments in Linda Dyson's book *Cervical Cancer* (see Bibliography).

Conserving the ovaries

Although most doctors do not now routinely remove ovaries during a hysterectomy, they frequently remove the ovaries in menopausal or post-menopausal women. If there is no disease in the ovaries, once again, there is no real justification for this. The rationale doctors use is that the ovaries cease working at menopause. This is not entirely true. The ovaries slow down, but do not shut down at menopause. They might produce some oestrogen for another 20 years and we need oestrogen to keep our vaginas elastic and healthy, and to prevent osteoporosis, a disease in which the bones lose density, leading to crippling and sometimes fatal fractures.

The other argument is that the development of ovarian cancer can be prevented by taking the ovaries out. However, this must be placed in perspective. Ovarian cancer is not common and the chance of a woman who has had a hysterectomy developing it is no greater, but we don't argue that all women should have their ovaries removed to prevent them getting cancer!

The loss of oestrogen if the ovaries are removed might also decrease the woman's risk of developing breast cancer, as breast cancer is linked to oestrogen. When young women have their ovaries removed, it is important that they have oestrogen replacement therapy or they will be plunged into a sudden and severe menopause, called a surgical menopause. This would put them at additional risk of osteoporosis, said to be around 50 percent.

Vaginal vs abdominal hysterectomy

The uterus can be removed in two ways:

- Abdominally, by cutting through the skin and muscle either vertically or horizontally. Horizontal cuts are usually made near the top of the pubic hair, called a 'bikini cut'. There will be stitches in the abdomen and the top of the vagina.
- Vaginally, through the top of the vagina. The vagina walls are held open by an instrument and the doctor cuts the uterus away between the cervix and vaginal vault. There are no external stitches, but there are stitches at the top of the vagina.

There are different factors to weigh up in deciding which type of operation is right, and your doctor will advise you which is preferable for you. Not all hysterectomies can be performed vaginally. Abdominal surgery is always performed in the following situations:

- If there is cancer.
- If the uterus is very big and bulky because of fibroids or some other cause. During a vaginal hysterectomy, the uterus is pulled downwards. If it is too big it cannot be pulled down.
- If there is infection or adhesions from previous operations (such as Caesarian section) gluing the uterus in position. In general, if there is infection or disease, the doctor needs to look at the tubes and ovaries.
- If endometriosis is present. The doctor will want to remove other cysts in the pelvic cavity.
- If there is any suggestion of disease in the ovaries it is not easy to remove the ovaries by the vaginal route, so an abdominal hysterectomy must be performed. The fact that the ovaries are not usually removed during the vaginal operation will, of course, protect the woman against their casual removal.

Most vaginal hysterectomies are performed on women with pelvic relaxation or prolapse. They are also preferred for obese women.

There are differing views among doctors about vaginal hysterectomy. Some say that women who have had their uterus removed vaginally recover more quickly. In an informal study at Middlemore Hospital, Professor Colin Mantell found that the average stay in hospital for abdominal hysterectomies was 8.4 days; for vaginal hysterectomies the average was 6.7 days. He pointed out that in interpreting these figures we need to take into account the fact that all patients with cancer will have had abdominal surgery, although all cervical cancer cases go to National Women's Hospital.

Professor Hutton prefers vaginal hysterectomies, saying that the operation time is shorter (30–45 minutes for vaginal; 45–90 minutes for abdominal), there is less sickness and nausea, and there is only one lot of stitches to heal. Women who have had a vaginal hysterectomy are usually able to move about earlier, as they don't have any pain from an abdominal wound. This helps prevent blood clots.

There have been suggestions that there is a higher rate of infection after vaginal hysterectomy, and urinary tract infection is clearly more frequent after a vaginal operation. But a study published in the *New England Medical Journal* in 1982 showed that there was actually less infection at the wound site in the vagina than at the abdominal wound site. Because in vaginal hysterectomy the operation site is close to the ureter and bladder, infections are quite common and injuries occasionally occur. Ureteral injuries, although rare (estimated to be around one in 1 000 of all hysterectomies), can be serious and are more likely to occur during vaginal surgery. During abdominal hysterectomy there is less chance of injuring these structures, because there is more direct vision, and it is easier to see that damage has inadvertently been done.

There is general agreement that there is more risk of both

immediate and delayed haemorrhage after a vaginal hysterectomy. It usually occurs after the vaginal packing is removed.

Enterocele, where the intestines bulge into the vagina, can occur after vaginal hysterectomy and, very rarely, part of the Fallopian tube can be caught in the scar tissue at the vaginal vault. Some writers, such as Vicki Hufnagel, have said that the vagina can be shortened by vaginal hysterectomy, resulting in problems with intercourse, and a few of our respondents felt that this had happened to them. Vaginal prolapse (the top of the vagina falling down) is thought to be more common with vaginal hysterectomy, although it is nevertheless still unusual.

Research in Canada has shown that women who have abdominal hysterectomies on average visited the doctor 7.3 times in the year after surgery, compared with 6.3 visits for women operated on vaginally. The normal population visit rate was 4.4.

There is an increasing preference on the part of surgeons and many women for vaginal hysterectomy where it is possible, although 1985 New Zealand hospital figures show that abdominal hysterectomy (4142) is still more frequent than vaginal (2091).

Most writers on the subject warn that the vaginal method requires practice and skill. You may want to check your surgeon's experience with this method. Specialist consultants in teaching or large women's hospitals will probably possess the necessary skills. Older private gynaecologists or young doctors in training may have had less practice. Asking a doctor how often he or she has performed a particular operation may be a touchy subject (for the doctor), but one that is important to us, and therefore worth asking about. We wouldn't take a Jaguar to a motor mechanic who specialised in Morris Minors, or vice versa. We do have a right to know our doctors' credentials before they take up the scalpel.

Getting prepared

In our survey, women were asked how they felt at the time of the operation. Twenty-nine percent replied that they felt unprepared for it.

You can prepare yourself for your operation before you even enter hospital. Many factors will affect how well you cope with the operation and recovery. There are some things you can do nothing about, such as your age, but you do have some control over other aspects of your life. The healthier you are before the operation, the less it will knock you back. So eating sensibly, stopping smoking, getting fit and having plenty of rest will improve your chances of a good recovery.

Smokers have more chance of suffering a blot clot or contracting a chest infection after surgery, and coughing while you have stitches is unpleasant. If you are taking oestrogen, for example, in oral contraceptives, it is advisable to stop these about two months before any surgery, because of the risk of a blood clot. You would have to use some other form of contraception, such as condoms. The doctor may advise you to lose weight because excess weight increases the risk of blood clot, or you may need iron or blood transfusions if you are severely anaemic. If your health has run down because of prolonged heavy bleeding it may be difficult, however, to do much about getting ready except take plenty of rest.

One woman who answered our hysterectomy questionnaire was a staff nurse who had worked in a gynaecology ward. She had some advice for women facing hysterectomy.

> I would like to see every woman advised to stop smoking as soon as she goes on the waiting list and told of the importance of physical fitness. She should be urged to start a walking regime that she can take up again once she is convalescent. I feel very strongly she should be told to walk daily for twenty minutes at a rate to get up a gentle sweat. She should be advised to get used to drinking about eight large glasses of water each day and the post-op fluid push would not seem so awful.

Read your consent form carefully. If you are adamant you want your ovaries retained, write it in. You can discuss beforehand what you would like done if by some chance a more severe condition requiring extensive surgery is discovered once the doctor has started operating. You can choose whether to leave it up to the doctor or be woken up to make your own decision.

Many consent forms in New Zealand hospitals are woefully inadequate, virtually giving the doctor *carte blanche*. In the aftermath of the Cervical Cancer Inquiry most hospitals are revising their consent forms. They should say precisely what the operation consists of, what will be removed or altered, who will do the operation, and specify any other matters, such as the presence of students. Even in a teaching hospital you can insist on knowing the name of the doctor who is to perform the operation; indeed, you should have met and discussed the operation with that doctor.

If there is anything special you want the staff to do, such as show you the uterus when it is removed or to take it when you leave the hospital, discuss this beforehand.

In hospital

Going into hospital is quite an experience, especially for women who have never been sick before. Some women enjoy being cared for by other people, while others resent losing their independence. Being a patient means having to fit in with hospital routines. How rigidly the rules are enforced depends on individual members of staff: some are more flexible than others. The trend now is towards creating a more home-like atmosphere where the patient is seen not as an inanimate object, but as someone whose wishes should be taken into consideration. Yet even if the staff are sympathetic it is easy to feel powerless in this strange new environment.

Before being admitted you should have seen the surgeon several times and should have had adequate time to find out why a hysterectomy has been recommended, and to make the decision without feeling pressured. The surgeon may have asked you to sign the written consent form at the last appointment before admission. If this has not happened you must sign the consent form in hospital.

We talked to Jill Bonham, a charge nurse at National Women's Hospital in Auckland, Dr Paul Hutchison, an Auckland gynaecologist who also works at National Women's Hospital, and Professor John Hutton, of Wellington Hospital, about hospital procedure for hysterectomy. The procedure outlined here largely follows what happens at National Women's Hospital. There will be some variations in procedure in different hospitals, but it should be broadly similar.

Admission to hospital

You will be asked to visit a pre-admitting clinic about a week before surgery. At this, you will have your health very thoroughly checked, which is always important before an operation, and tests, including blood and urine tests, will be done. Checks for anaesthetic risk, asthma, heart, lungs and nutritional status should also be made. The results of these tests will be available when you come in to hospital for the operation.

These days women quite often go in to hospital in the morning and have their surgery in the afternoon, but some doctors still prefer their patients to be admitted on the previous day. The time of admission is something you should negotiate with the surgeon, and your point of view should be taken into account.

When you arrive at the hospital there is an admitting procedure that has to be followed, and there will be forms to fill in. After completing these you will be shown to the ward. In many hospitals a special nurse will be assigned to you and this nurse will be the staff member you will get to know best during your stay in hospital. She will probably take you around the ward on arrival and show you where everything is. She should give you a copy of the Patients' Code of Rights. She should tell you about any drips, drains and catheters you will wake up with after the operation, and be able to answer any questions you have about what will happen before, during and after the surgery. It is part of her job to provide emotional support too. There is more emphasis these days on a holistic approach to nursing and some nurses are also happy to use techniques such as massage, and are more open about alternative medicine than they used to be.

On the day of surgery there is usually a pre-operative nursing check, which you will be asked to sign. The nurse may also be required to do a written nursing care assessment. This assessment will include some comments about your expectations while in hospital and a social and psychological assessment. If you want to see what has been written about you, feel free to ask. The nurse may ask you to make your own comments or to check that everything that has been recorded about you is true and fair.

During these few hours before surgery you may like to have a partner or friend to keep you company. There should be no problem about this, although it would be courteous to check this out beforehand.

There are some things that have to be done before surgery that most women thoroughly dislike. Pubic shaves are still done in some hospitals as a guard against infection. Sometimes only a partial shave will be done or the hair clipped. A small enema or suppository may also be required to ensure that the bowel is empty before the operation. You will usually be given prophylactic antibiotics to prevent infection. This most often is a single dose of antibiotic given intravenously just before surgery. Sometimes the antibiotic is continued for 24 hours.

The anaesthetist will visit you before the operation to again check your suitability for the anaesthetic, and will be able to explain what anaesthetic is to be used, what his or her job is during the operation, and how you can expect to feel afterwards. The surgeon, or another member of the medical team, will also visit and be available for information.

Shortly before going down to surgery you will be offered an oral pre-medication, which will make you feel relaxed and drowsy, and you will be asked to change from your own clothes into a theatre gown. When all the formalities are over, and you are ready, you will be wheeled down to theatre in your own bed.

In theatre

On arrival in theatre you will be met by theatre nursing staff. Your name and the kind of operation you are having will be double-checked by the theatre staff and they will also make sure that your signature is on the consent form.

The operation is usually done under a full anaesthetic, although you may have chosen to have it done with an epidural anaesthetic. For a general anaesthetic the anaesthetist will come and give you an intravenous injection of anaesthetic, usually in one of the veins in the back of your hand. This will put you to sleep almost immediately.

The anaesthetist will then insert a small tube down your throat into the trachea. At the end of this is a small bag which, when it is inflated, stops any food from the stomach from getting into the lungs. If any particles still manage to get past, bubbles appear and the debris can be sucked up through the tube so the passage is cleared.

You will now be connected to a life support system. This consists of a machine that systematically pumps air and anaesthetic gases in and out of your lungs, an electrocardiograph machine and a blood-pressure machine. This life support system gives a continuous printout of your blood pressure, pulse and heartbeat throughout the operation. Any problem shows up at once and staff can take immediate action to put things right.

First your legs will be placed in stirrups. A nurse will now empty your bladder with a catheter and Bonney's blue antiseptic will be painted on your vagina to cleanse and sterilise it. Sterile

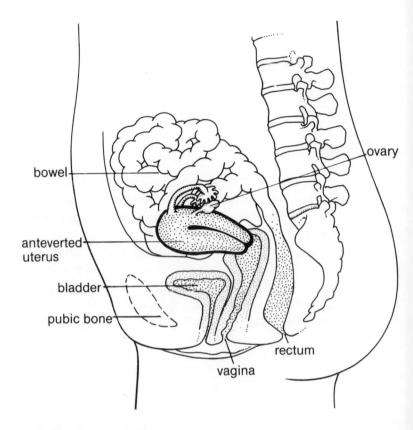

bowel

ovary

anteverted uterus

bladder

pubic bone

rectum

vagina

Before hysterectomy.

cloth will be draped over your body.

If you are having a vaginal hysterectomy the surgeon will remove the cervix and uterus through the top of the vagina. The cervix will be grasped with an instrument and an incision made right around it. The bladder will be pushed up out of the way and then the uterus and the cervix will be cut away, including the ligaments that support the uterus. The ovaries will be left in place. The uterus and cervix will be pulled down through the vagina and removed whole. The surgeon will examine the uterus carefully

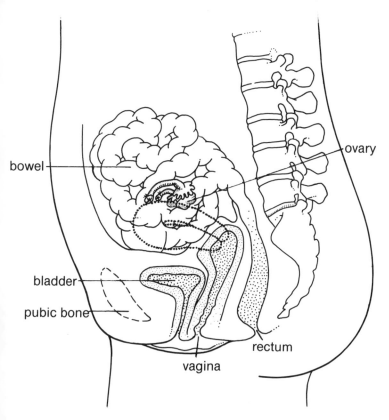

bowel

ovary

bladder

pubic bone

rectum

vagina

After hysterectomy.

The top of the vagina is closed off and the bowel moves into the space where the uterus has been. The ends of the Fallopian tubes have been clamped off during surgery and the ovaries remain in their original position.

and it will then be sent to the laboratory for a more detailed inspection.

The major ligaments will be sewn together to give support to the top of the vagina and the vaginal tissue will be sewn up at the top, re-forming a normally sized and shaped vagina.

A catheter may be left within the bladder until you are mobile, in order to prevent trauma to the urethra. Some surgeons leave a pack in the vagina to stem bleeding.

If you are having abdominal hysterectomy the surgeon will first make an incision across the stomach. Your body will then be tilted head down so that gravity pulls the intestine and bowel out of the way, allowing the surgeon to see and feel inside the abdomen more easily.

A sterile pad may be put inside the abdomen to keep the intestine to one side. Clamps will now be put onto the round ligament, Fallopian tubes and suspensory ligaments on either side of the uterus. These structures will then be tied. The uterus will be pulled up and the bladder pulled forward. A cut will be made between the bladder and the uterus, pushing the bladder out of the way. Clamps will then be put on the uterine arteries, and the arteries will be cut and tied. The cervix will now be freed from the top of the vagina and cut away and removed with the uterus. If it is necessary the ovaries and/or Fallopian tubes can also be removed at this point. The surgeon will examine the uterus and send it to the laboratory.

The vagina will now be stitched at the top. At this point the surgeon will take the opportunity to check out that all is well inside and take a look at other body organs, such as the bowel, liver and stomach. Before closing the abdomen there will be a check to make sure that any bleeding where stitches have been put in is not excessive. The surgeon will then stitch up the abdomen.

While this is happening the theatre staff will make a thorough tally to make sure that all the instruments and swabs used during the operation have been removed.

A small polythene drain tube will be inserted as the abdomen is being closed. This allows the slight bleeding which will still be taking place to drain away, thus preventing festering.

Once the sewing up is finished the anaesthetic will be reversed and you will start to breathe normally again. The tube will be removed from your throat and you will be taken to the recovery room.

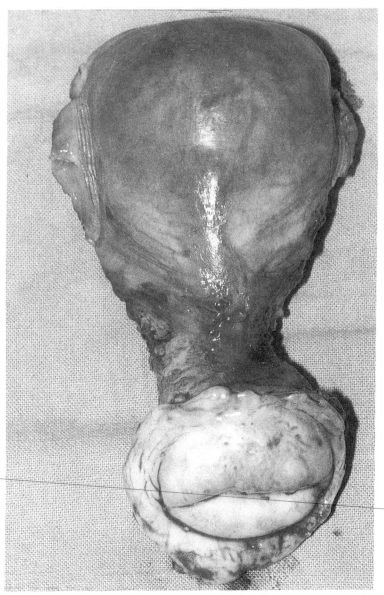

A cervix and uterus after removal during hysterectomy. The uterus is usually 7.5-9.5 cm long.

After surgery

A nurse will stay with you in the recovery room until you regain consciousness. Depending on how heavily you are anaesthetised you may wake up almost immediately, or not for an hour or so. When you do wake up you will be taken back to the ward. But, although you are technically awake, you may not be aware of what is going on and may drift in and out of consciousness for some time.

The intravenous drip that was inserted in theatre will be left in for a day or so to give extra fluid. This will supply fluids if nausea makes drinking difficult. The catheter may also be left in place to make sure that the bladder starts to work well after the operation, because the operation area is very close to the bladder and can affect its working. There may also be a drainage tube from the vagina or the abdomen to drain away excess blood. This blood must come away to allow healing to take place.

It is not unusual to feel nauseous at first, and this may last up to 24 hours. Nausea is more likely after an abdominal hysterectomy, because the gut is moved out of the way to get to the uterus, and this can cause feelings of gut disturbance. Nausea can also be a reaction to the anaesthetic and to the drugs given for pain relief. Sucking ice, sips of water and breathing exercises can help. If it persists anti-emetic drugs may help.

The amount of pain women experience after a hysterectomy varies greatly. Some women have a much higher pain threshold than others. Some women are nervous about pain relief injections and others are stoical and say they don't need them. This is fine except for those women who then find that every little movement hurts so much that they lie very still to minimise the pain. It is very important to start moving again after the operation, because it decreases the likelihood of blood clots forming, so it is often better to have some pain relief in the early stages.

One of the things that women are not always warned about before they go into hospital is how their bowels may be affected.

One of the main topics of conversation in a gynaecological ward is wind. After surgery the gut motion may slow down for a while, and it is a fact of life that gases tend to build up in an inactive bowel. This happens to most women. The physiotherapist will give advice about what to do about this. Pelvic tilting, exercises and being out of bed and moving around can help. Some hospitals can provide a special wind cocktail.

If you have not had a bowel motion by day three a suppository will probably be handed out to help things along. But often this won't be necessary. You should be able to pass urine on your own, but if there is a problem you may be given a catheter.

Coping with drips, drains and catheters, and trying to get the body to function normally again after the hysterectomy is a big effort, so visitors are a welcome distraction. A hysterectomy is, however, major surgery and on the first day it is probably wise to have only one special visitor who won't mind a rather sleepy patient. On the following days most women enjoy more visitors, provided they don't turn up in droves and stay for hours on end. But it is really good to have friends who care.

Emotional support is especially important on the third day, when many women experience a reaction similar to the baby blues. Women who were feeling positive and coping well will often dissolve mysteriously into tears on this day, and will welcome some tender loving care. It may just be a reaction to having an operation, or it may be the day when the finality of the operation sinks in.

I remember the day after having had the operation I had a dream. The lady in the bed next to me was called Ivy. Well I dreamt that I had a very little baby (about the size of Tom Thumb) and it was sitting among an ivy vine, covering the wall of a house. When I tried to pick up my baby I could not find it any more. When I woke up I realised for the first time that I would never have a baby again. So it must have had some mental effect on me at the time, although I have never looked back since then. I found that a positive attitude helped a lot.

Women are expected to be up and about very quickly these days. If the operation was in the morning you may be helped to get up that evening, or at the very latest on the next day. That evening you might try a short walk and the next day you should be able to have a shower. The main reason for getting women up so soon is that activity will prevent thrombosis in the legs.

The surgeon who did the operation should call in either on the evening of the day on which the operation was done, and he or she (or another member of the team if it is a public hospital) should visit every day. The surgeon should explain at an early stage what he or she found during the operation and which organs were removed. Some hospitals have a sheet of paper with a diagram of that part of the body. If this is not available the surgeon should be asked to find some paper and to draw a diagram showing what has been removed.

Throughout your stay in hospital you should make good use of the nurse who has been assigned to you. Feel free to ask her any questions and get some emotional support too. Many women cope well in hospital but those who don't should not feel they are abnormal. Public hospitals have social workers available and you can ask to see one of them if you want. If you are unhappy about the way you are being treated, there will probably be a patient advocate in the hospital whom you can ask to see.

It is sometimes difficult to know which questions to ask the nurse and which to ask the surgeon. If in doubt ask both. No questions should be left unanswered.

The hospital stay will be about five days, unless there are complications, which is not at all unusual. The most common complications are infections and bowel and bladder problems.

On the last day before going home the stitches are usually taken out. The surgeon may have used ordinary sutures, dissolving sutures, clips or staples. Their removal can sometimes be a bit uncomfortable. Some women leave hospital after only three days. This is too early to have stitches removed, and they will usually go back to their own GP to have this done.

Before you leave hospital make sure you have all the information you need about what you can and can't do when you get home, and whom to contact if you are worried about anything. If there are any problems before the six-weekly check-up you can ring and ask the hospital for advice, but it is often more convenient to ring your GP, especially if you live some distance from the hospital. The GP can then arrange for your re-admission to hospital if necessary. Of course if you are a private patient you can ring your own gynaecologist. Most women won't need to have further medical attention, apart from the six-weekly check-up to make sure that everything has healed well. They should have an uneventful recovery and look forward to feeling fit and well again.

9

COMPLICATIONS AND NEGATIVE EFFECTS OF HYSTERECTOMY

Hysterectomy is very safe surgery, with a low death rate. A recent statistical profile from New York State reported that where hysterectomy was the main operation, the death rate was 2.5 per 1 000 patients. Most of the deaths were in cancer-related cases. Excluding the cases that were cancer- or pregnancy-related, the death rate was 1.1 per 1 000.

The complication rate from hysterectomy is quite high — 40 percent of cases. Most complications are short-lived and not life-threatening. A 1983 study of hysterectomy in the United States by the American College of Obstetrics and Gynaecology and the Department of Health and Human Services concluded that 'one-fourth to one-half of all women who undergo hysterectomy develop some morbidity [disease] with fever and haemorrhage the most common type'.

A Canadian study showed that complications serious enough to require hospital re-admission occurred at a rate of 3.7 percent after abdominal hysterectomy and 4.8 percent after vaginal hysterectomy. An Australian study showed that 7.4 percent of the women surveyed required re-admission.

In our survey 64 percent of women reported having one or more negative effects. Only 4 percent of women reported solely negative effects, while 35 percent reported only positive ones. Sixty percent reported both positive and negative effects, while 7 women experienced neither.

The main problems noted by women in our survey were depression (31 percent), hot flushes (29 percent), bladder and bowel problems (28 percent), mood swings (26 percent), less satisfactory sex life (20 percent), infection (15 percent), difficulty experiencing orgasm (14 percent), feeling incomplete as a woman (13 percent), grief at loss of fertility (13 percent) and haemorrhage (7 percent). It is possible that women would not have been told if a haemorrhage had occurred while they were under anaesthetic.

For all the negative effects, the number of respondents who received treatment was low. For example, only 29 percent of women who were depressed and 35 percent of those with bladder and bowel problems received help. This lack of assistance was especially noticeable for women who had sexual problems. We don't know from our survey whether women sought help but did not find it, or whether they just put up with their problems. If you have any difficulties, get help from your doctor, a counsellor or a women's group. We hope that this book will also help women find their own ways of coping, by assisting them in understanding the causes of negative effects. Being able to put names on problems and getting understandable explanations helps with dealing with them. Not knowing the truth can lead to self-blame and a feeling that your life is out of control.

To put the risks and possible negative effects of hysterectomy in perspective, it is important to also talk about the positive benefits women reported. Eighty-four percent of the women reported relief of their symptoms, and 83 percent were pleased not to have periods. In fact, in our survey only 3 percent of the women regretted no longer menstruating. Given that so many women had such problems with heavy bleeding, this is not surprising!

The emphasis in the following list of negative effects is on those with a direct physical cause. Depression and sexual problems are examined in more detail in separate chapters.

Thromboembolism (blot clots)
There is a risk of thrombosis or blood clot in a vein because the

woman's legs are stationary for some time during the operation and may be lifted in the air. This can stop blood flowing through veins and promote clot formation during or after surgery. At Wellington Hospital some women are given the anti-coagulant Heparin to make the blood more fluid, although this increases the chance of bleeding at the wound site. Alternatively, special stockings may be put on the legs to aid circulation. In some hospitals the legs are massaged during surgery. Walking and moving round as soon as possible after surgery helps prevent clots. Symptoms of a thrombosis are slight fever, tenderness in the calves or swelling of an ankle.

Lung problems

Lung infections and pneumonia can occur because of the anaesthetic, especially in smokers and asthmatics. A physiotherapist may help you with exercises before and after the operation. Breathing exercises and body movements help lessen the risk. Antibiotics are now almost routinely given and this has dramatically reduced the incidence of lung and other infections.

Haemorrhage

Haemorrhage during the operation is not uncommon and blood transfusions are not infrequently given during hysterectomy surgery (8–19 percent of operations). Haemorrhage can also occur after surgery, while the woman is in hospital or occasionally after leaving hospital. This is one reason for getting back into normal activities, including sexual intercourse, gradually.

Haematoma

A few women who filled in our questionnaire reported developing a painful haematoma or internal bruise at the incision site, either in the abdomen or at the top of the vagina. This can sometimes be drained, but often must be simply left to dissipate, which can take many weeks.

Wound infection

Infections at the wound site are quite common after hysterectomy. The wound site becomes red and painful and pus may discharge from it. The woman can become hot and fevered. The usual treatment is antibiotics, although the doctor may sometimes decide to drain it. Occasionally a wound will burst open from infection and need to be restitched.

Bladder problems

Bladder problems and infections are quite common after hysterectomy. The bladder is very close to the uterus and may be bruised during surgery. Women quite frequently need a catheter in the bladder after surgery to help get urination going again. Cystitis, which causes pain during urination and a constant feeling of wanting to pass water, will be treated with antibiotics.

If a bladder repair has been carried out in conjunction with the hysterectomy, then a catheter that comes out above the pubic bone will be inserted during surgery and left in place until the woman is moving around. This is to avoid trauma to the urethra by frequent catheterisation and to prevent any bladder infection.

Sometimes the bladder will not function to its former level of efficiency in the weeks or months following surgery. Women report infections and leaking urine, especially if they cough or jump. The bladder will usually gradually regain its competence, but such symptoms can indicate a more serious complication and should always be reported to a doctor.

Research in Canada has shown that in the first year after surgery women who have had hysterectomies make twice as many visits to the doctor for urinary tract infections as cholecystectomy (removal of gallbladder) patients and three times as many as the female population in general. By the second year, this differential has narrowed although post-hysterectomy patients still have more visits. American research has shown that while women visit their doctors less frequently with gynaecological problems after surgery, they visit more frequently with urinary tract infections, psychological problems and menopausal symptoms.

Prevention of recurrent cystitis can be assisted by care in sexual intercourse. Make sure you are properly aroused and lubricated before penetration. Empty the bladder immediately after sex, carefully wash the genitals and drink several glasses of water. Preparations for keeping the urine alkaline can be bought from the chemist (Citravescent or Ural) or prescribed by the doctor. Especially troublesome cystitis might call for preventative drug treatment, such as a big dose of an appropriate drug, for example, Amoxil, after intercourse, especially if it has been vigorous. Women with persistent bladder problems should drink a lot of water and avoid coffee, tea and alcohol.

Bladder injuries

The ureters are the tubes that run from the kidneys to the bladder. Occasionally, in about one in a thousand hysterectomies, one of the ureters is cut during surgery. If it is detected at the time, it will be rejoined or replanted in the bladder. If it is not, fluid cannot get through into the bladder and may leak into the abdominal cavity. Symptoms are fever, pain and distension of the abdomen. If it is not detected, the kidneys can be affected. Further surgery will be necessary to repair the damage. In New Zealand one woman successfully gained compensation for the loss of a kidney after a hysterectomy. In this case the surgeon failed to take action for some months after the woman reported problems and the kidney was damaged beyond repair. Injury to the ureter can cause lifelong urinary problems.

It is also possible for a hole to be poked in the bladder during surgery. The risk of this is estimated to be about 1 in 500. If it is recognised at the time, a repair can be made during surgery; if it is not, the problem will emerge afterwards, with urine leaking through a hole between the bladder and the top of the vagina. Sometimes resting the bladder will allow this hole, called a fistula, to heal. If it will not heal, repair surgery must be performed. This requires a very skilled surgeon.

Bowel problems

The bowel is also close to the uterus and it can be affected by surgery. It takes a while to get going again after the operation, so food and fluid intake will be restricted for about 24 hours after the operation. Once the woman starts eating, she may get some pain as the bowel starts working, while the mechanism that empties the bowel has not yet returned to normal. Passing wind will help the pain, and is quite normal after a hysterectomy. Painkillers can be given, and sometimes staff will suggest a laxative or enema. One woman told us that a nurse got her to lie on her side and massage her stomach and this helped to relieve the pain.

Occasionally the bowel can be temporarily paralysed after surgery. In such cases, the woman will be given intravenous feeding by fluid until the bowel recovers. Constipation after surgery can be relieved by eating a high fibre diet, and wind will be minimised by avoiding foods such as onions, cabbage, Brussels sprouts, turnips, swedes, legumes (beans) and spicy food.

Very occasionally a hole can be made in the bowel during surgery and a repair operation is necessary. Bowel obstructions can also occur if scar tissue closes the bowel.

Failure to heal

Sometimes the tissue at the top of the vagina fails to heal in the usual time. It may discharge or bleed and cause pain during intercourse. The usual treatment for this is an application of silver nitrate, or cautery of the area.

Nerve injury

Sometimes nerves, especially the femoral nerve in the leg, can be damaged by instruments used in the surgery. This can cause numbness in the thigh and leg, instability of the knee and pain. This will usually mend itself over time. Serious nerve injury is very rare and would require neurological attention.

Prolapse

While hysterectomy is frequently performed for various types of gynaecological prolapse, after hysterectomy it is still possible for remaining organs to prolapse, or sag down into the vagina. The walls of the vagina can collapse inwards or the top fall down. This is most likely to occur in an elderly woman whose hysterectomy was performed because of prolapse. Repairing such injuries can be difficult without damaging the vagina.

Vaginal injuries

Where the hysterectomy is performed because of a vaginal prolapse such as cystocele (sagging bladder or supports under bladder) or rectocele (bowel) the surgeon will also repair the vagina, cutting away excess skin — in essence, taking a tuck in the vagina. A certain amount of physician judgement comes into play here and the doctor may act on a very personal view of what is needed. If this is not discussed previously with the woman, she may find that her vagina has been 'remade' into a size or shape not comfortable for her. The vagina may be too narrow or short and intercourse may cause considerable pain. One woman who was 35 at the time of her operation told us:

> During my post-op visit to the surgeon I was stunned when he informed me that during surgery he had 'tightened up the vagina', which would please my husband. Attempts at intercourse following the surgery failed due to the excruciating pain I experienced. The cause was either too narrow an entry or painful scarring. We persevered for some considerable time but the condition did not improve. The result is that we no longer indulge in intercourse at all.

She felt so betrayed by the surgeon that she could not return to him, even when advised to do so by a sex therapist.

Women who have radiotherapy for cancer suffer more complications than other hysterectomy patients. The vaginal tissue may be so damaged by the radiotherapy that it loses its elasticity and penetration is painful. Sometimes using dilators to stretch the tissues can help, but women who have had radiotherapy do report continuing sexual problems. They are also more likely to suffer fistulas between the bowel or bladder and these are very difficult to repair because the tissue is damaged.

Problems with the scar

It is quite normal for the scar in an abdominal hysterectomy to itch or sting as it is healing and nerve endings are growing back. However, some women have continuing pain in the scar and others report they have a pot belly or the scar is unsightly. One woman wrote: 'My body shape has changed. I have always had a flat stomach except during pregnancy. Now I have a fixed belly which I find awkward and uncomfortable. I feel the scar has created a ledge.'

According to the British gynaecologist Dr Wendy Savage, this is caused by fat necrosis, or fat dying because it has been cut during surgery. One way of avoiding it is to lose weight before surgery and have firm stomach muscles. The stomach sagging, Dr Savage says, usually follows an infection in the wound. Physiotherapy could help with this problem.

Menstrual and menopausal symptoms

Removing the uterus will stop periods, but it will not usually stop the other symptoms of our menstrual cycle. The ovaries still go through their cycle so signs of hormonal changes, such as swollen breasts, bloating and premenstrual tension, may still be there. Some women report an improvement in these symptoms, others report worsening.

Normally menopause occurs at the time it would have anyway, with all the same symptoms, except for loss of periods. There has been little research on whether hysterectomy affects women's experience of the menopause, although a recent Massachusetts study showed that women who have a surgical menopause through removal of ovaries have the hardest time with menopausal symptoms, despite hormone replacement therapy.

Hot flushes, depression and sexual problems

Significant numbers of our respondents reported depression, hot flushes, mood swings, less satisfactory sex lives and difficulty reaching orgasm after hysterectomy.

There can be a number of causes for these problems and some are related to our feelings of self-esteem. But these symptoms can also be caused by the effect on the ovaries of removal of the uterus.

Hot flushes are a menopausal symptom. Depression, mood swings, loss of libido and enjoyment of sex can also be menopausal symptoms. During the menopause the hormones are unstable as oestrogen production slows down. The vagina can also become less elastic and lubricate less or more slowly.

Women are told to expect menopausal symptoms if their ovaries are removed during the hysterectomy operation. If the women are younger than menopausal age they will probably routinely be given hormone replacement therapy (HRT) to offset the loss of oestrogen.

However, the prevailing medical wisdom has been that if the ovaries are not removed, or if one is removed, or even if only part of one ovary is retained, menopausal symptoms are impossible because the remaining ovary or ovaries will be sufficient to maintain oestrogen production.

Consequently, when women who still have their ovaries have reported hot flushes, they have often been disbelieved or told that this is a natural menopause occurring coincidentally. In our survey, women in their twenties reported hot flushes after hysterectomy, which makes the possibility of a coincidental menopause extremely remote.

> I think the fact that I had only just had my twenty-ninth birthday made it seem as if I had grown 'old' overnight. I still have my ovaries but it seems to have interfered hormonally and I still have hot flushes.

If women have had emotional effects, such as depression or mood swings, the argument has been that they were psychologically unstable before the operation, that they were depressed about losing their fertility, or that they have suffered a blow to their self-esteem. Often women who complain of depression have been prescribed anti-depressants.

It has also been argued that depression can occur after any major surgery. Some men, the argument goes, become depressed after coronary surgery.

Doctors have observed over many years the relative frequency with which women become depressed after hysterectomy and so there has been a good deal of research in this area. However, much of it has been poorly designed and the results are conflicting. The Oxford research of D. Gath and others was, however, very carefully designed. These researchers interviewed women with heavy bleeding of benign origin 4 weeks before hysterectomy, then 6 and 18 months afterwards. They found that before surgery, 58 percent of the women were described as 'psychiatric cases'. Afterwards, this proportion reduced to 25.8 percent at 6 months, and 29 percent at 18 months. They concluded that hysterectomy seldom leads to psychiatric disorder and that many women have improved mental health.

Gath and other researchers have argued that women with psychiatric symptoms are more likely to end up having hysterectomies or gynaecological surgery in general. But it is also possible to argue that women become psychiatrically disturbed because of their physical problems and that removing those problems by hysterectomy will result in an improvement in their mental health. It is hardly surprising that women who have put up with pain and heavy, draining bleeding, who have worried about what to do about it, who have perhaps encountered unsympathetic doctors or waited for years on a surgery waiting list, and who have relationship or family problems as a result, will suffer emotionally in some way. And if the 'cause' is taken away, then many of those women could expect an improvement in their state of mind.

All sorts of explanations are given for some women's loss of sexual interest after hysterectomy. They weren't interested in sex anyway, and used their constant bleeding as a way of avoiding sex. Now their 'excuse' has been removed, they blame the operation for their frigidity. The 'normal' woman, it is argued, will be *more* interested in sex after hysterectomy because she won't fear pregnancy and won't have to cope with pain or messy bleeding any more.

Our survey showed that the women who had lost sexual interest were not relieved, but were clearly distressed about it. Only the very occasional woman was relieved to give up sex. This woman expressed the feeling of many:

> I was glad not to have the heavy bleeding, but after the relief from that I became sad that the closeness with one's partner which comes from having intercourse was gone. I was assured that my sex life would be 'heaps better', but it actually vanished. When I told the specialist we were having sexual difficulties, he said: 'It is all J's fault, he isn't taking time to turn you on' and that was that. I did try a couple of extramarital affairs but they were not really pleasing. I was unable to achieve orgasm ever again.

Some overseas researchers have not been so quick to dismiss such reports. As long ago as 1974 Dr D. H. Richards, writing in *The Lancet*, coined the term 'post-hysterectomy syndrome' for the results of his controlled trial, which showed high rates of hot flushes, tiredness, headaches, dizziness, loss of libido and insomnia (all symptoms of menopause) after hysterectomy. He found a depression rate of over 70 percent in hysterectomy patients, compared to 30 percent in his controls. Even excluding women in both groups who had had treatment for depression before the operation, he came up with the same ratio. Sixty-one percent of the women under 45 in whom one or both ovaries were preserved reported hot flushes. Oestrogen therapy, he said, helped some patients with loss of libido and some patients reported 'dramatic relief from depression'.

In another paper on this topic Dr Richards noted that the number of children a woman had made no difference to the incidence of depression. 'The effect of hysterectomy,' he wrote, 'seems in some respects to resemble that of menopause, but in an exaggerated form . . . [Hot flushes] and other symptoms raise the possibility that an endocrine factor may be involved even when the uterus alone is removed.'

More and more gynaecologists have come to accept that the removal of the uterus can by some unknown mechanism affect the functioning of the ovaries. Professor Mantell says that the blood supply to the ovaries may be damaged, causing some ovaries to not function as well. Professor Hutton agrees. The blood supply to the ovaries, he says, may be affected by the scar tissue that can form after surgery, or because the ovaries are drawn down during the operation.

There are other possible causes. We know that stress can stop periods; the stress of this major surgery could affect the ovaries as well. Professor Hutton says that the old idea that even part of an ovary was enough to supply adequate oestrogen production may not be correct. Each ovary may need the other to function well. If you remove one or part of one ovary, the other may not ovulate as well as before.

A paper in *The Lancet* in 1985 reported that in a percentage of women who have had their tubes tied, oestrogen production from the ovaries dropped significantly. This caused a disturbance in the oestrogen/progesterone ratio, which led to the heavy bleeding some women reported after sterilisation. The researcher postulated that a similar effect on hormones may be caused by removal of the uterus.

This uncertainty highlights the fact that we still do not know exactly what causes a hot flush. Dr Howard Judd of the University of California in Los Angeles has been researching the mechanism of the hot flush. So far, he has concluded that it is not removal of the ovary which causes it, but some as yet undiscovered hormonal mechanism involving other organs.

The results of our survey provided support for the belief that the ovaries are affected by hysterectomy. Sixty-three percent of the women who had uterus and both ovaries removed reported experiencing hot flushes, but so did 19 percent of the women who had only the uterus removed. Of the women who lost one ovary, 46 percent reported hot flushes. Other menopausal symptoms showed a similar pattern.

	Only uterus removed	Uterus & one ovary removed	Uterus & both ovaries removed
Hot flushes	19%	46%	63%
Depression	27%	36%	38%
Mood swings	23%	36%	33%
Difficulty reaching orgasm	11%	17%	21%
Less satisfactory sex life	16%	22%	32%

It should be remembered that apart from hot flushes, these symptoms cannot all be put down with certainty to hormonal causes. We can't really know what caused them in each individual woman. But it is interesting to note the pattern that emerged.

A percentage of women who did keep both their ovaries still described symptoms that could be menopausal. If one ovary was removed, the percentage increased. If both ovaries were removed, the percentage increased still further, except in the category of mood swings. This indicates that the ovaries can be affected by hysterectomy and that women's reports of menopausal symptoms after the operation should be taken seriously.

In her book *No More Hysterectomies* Vicki Hufnagel calls this effect 'ovary death', which may be a little dramatic. A more accurate description is probably ovarian failure. This is the term used by a group of West German researchers who conducted studies at Kiel University.

They reviewed the medical literature for research on this phenomenon and found that doctors have actually been reporting it since 1889. Thus doctors who currently deny it is possible are 100 years out-of-date!

The Kiel team said that previous studies had shown that ovarian failure occured in young women who had a hysterectomy with one or both ovaries retained in 25-50 percent of cases. They then conducted their own research involving 164 women, aged 27 to 42 years, who had had hysterectomies. Thirty-nine percent of the women reported menopausal symptoms after hysterectomy. The most frequently reported symptoms (nearly 40 percent) were hot flushes, weight gain, nervousness, and irritability (the women were not asked about sexual response). Around a quarter of the women also reported depression, insomnia, palpitations, headaches, vertigo and anxiety.

Women with only one ovary reported symptoms of ovarian failure more often than women with two. The incidence with one ovary was 52 percent, with two it was 37 percent. These proportions are consistent with our findings through our survey.

The West German team also undertook hormone studies on some of the women and found their oestrogen and progesterone levels were markedly lower than a group of non-hysterectomised women in the same age group.

These researchers believe that it may be interruption of the blood supply to the ovaries caused by the surgery which leads the ovaries to fail. They explain that the ovaries are supplied with blood by the ovarian artery and the uterine artery. The respective share these arteries take in feeding the ovaries varies considerably from woman to woman. Thus, the effect on the ovaries of hysterectomy will depend on the blood supply type of the woman. This explains why some women experience no effects while others do.

The West German team did not look at sexual response. But Vicki Hufnagel believes that ovarian failure may also account for some women's loss of sexual interest and capacity for orgasm after hysterectomy. Loss of oestrogen can also cause vaginal atrophy, vaginal dryness and therefore painful intercourse. The hormone testosterone is also produced by the ovaries and is essential to the sex drive of both men and women. Fifty percent of testosterone is produced by the ovaries; the other 50 percent is produced by the adrenal glands. Testosterone depletion, caused by inadequately functioning ovaries, could cause loss of libido.

The West German team concluded that because this ovarian failure is hormonally caused, what is needed by way of 'cure' is hormone replacement therapy, not the treatment for psychological problems so many women actually receive.

Testosterone can be replaced in several ways: by creams applied to the vagina, by monthly injections and by pellets implanted under the skin every 6–12 months. Oral tablets are not recommended because of the toxic effect on the liver. Testosterone has been very successful for some patients.

Unfortunately, it has only recently been recognised that some women might need replacement testosterone after the loss or failure of their ovaries, so there has been little research concerning safe doses, and there are quite a few problems. Testosterone can cause masculinising features, such as hair growth and deepening of the voice.

If ovarian failure is caused by stress or a temporary interruption of the blood supply, then the ovaries may regain their capacity with time. Menopausal symptoms would then lessen and disappear. Margaret Ryan's Australian research showed that 21 women (35 percent) had hot flushes after the surgery, but by 14 months after the operation only 3 women were experiencing them, although another 4 were by then on HRT.

While some women in our survey reported long-term symptoms, others said they did improve. The hot flushes dwindled, depression lifted, energy came back and sexual interest returned. Of course, this would only happen if there was an organic cause for the symptoms. If the cause is related to aspects of our lives, such as our feelings about ourselves and our relationships, the ovaries regaining their function will not be the answer.

Weight gain and hair growth

A small number of respondents to our questionnaire reported weight gain and thickening waistlines after hysterectomy, although we had not asked about this. Conversely, one woman described losing two inches from her waist after a huge fibroid was removed along with her uterus.

Margaret Ryan, in her Australian research, found that 43 percent of the women she studied gained 3.5 kg or more after hysterectomy.

It has been usual in the past to dismiss these reports from women as old wives' tales. The explanation, we have been told, is lack of exercise after the operation and normal ageing. It *is* normal for women to gain weight and spread around the waist as they age, so it is difficult to isolate the actual cause for these reports from women. But if women can suffer some loss of ovarian function after hysterectomy, it is also possible to argue that this might be the cause.

The same can be said for facial hair growth, which a very few women reported in our survey. Maybe it was going to happen anyway, but we can't dismiss the idea that diminished ovarian function could be a cause.

Hormone replacement therapy

Hormone replacement therapy (HRT) is usually given to pre-menopausal women who have lost their ovaries, unless there is a contraindication, such as a prior disease aggravated by oestrogen, for example, endometriosis or ovarian cancer. These women are especially at risk of osteoporosis from early loss of oestrogen.

In the past, most HRT used only oestrogen. In the seventies huge numbers of American women were given this therapy as a kind of youth elixir. It was then found that the oestrogen caused increased rates of endometrial cancer and the therapy fell into disrepute. Now HRT is coming into fashion again, this time with the addition of progestin, an artificial progesterone, for part of the cycle, to get around the cancer risk.

Of course, women who have had the uterus removed cannot get endometrial cancer and the progestin may not strictly be necessary for them. Nevertheless, some doctors writing about HRT think even women who have had hysterectomies should get progestin because there is some evidence that this may decrease the risk of cancer of the breast. On the other hand, other doctors worry that progestin may *increase* the risk of breast cancer.

Although there have been numerous studies on oestrogen therapy, there has been much less on HRT containing progestin. Dr P. C. MacDonald, an American endocrinologist, wrote in the *New England Medical Journal* that we just don't know the long-term risk of HRT. He reminded readers that it was only after many years that the hazards of combined oestrogen and progestin in the Pill became apparent. He recommended caution with HRT.

Several of our respondents wrote about the difference hormone replacement therapy made to their post-hysterectomy symptoms.

> I still feel pleased about the repair, but angry I had to put up with depression, mood swings and an unsatisfactory and painful sex life for over three years before I took the matter into my own hands and saw a specialist without my doctor's knowledge. I have been prescribed oestrogen replacement, which my doctor is not happy about, but my specialist says I can stay on it for the rest of my life. What a difference!

Another woman wrote:

> After my hysterectomy and because I didn't have my ovaries

removed, I shouldn't by rights need oestrogen therapy. So for a year I lay around lifeless, depressed, no interest in anything. In the end I went to my local doctor because I was always so tired. He most certainly didn't understand and more or less told me I was a bit crazy and to go home and pull myself together, which was so terrible. Getting desperate I rang my specialist, who had me come in and see him. He put me on oestrogen. Just about overnight I was back to my old self. The shock of the operation had stopped my ovaries working. After oestrogen therapy for about three years, I'm back to normal and don't need it any more.

Hormone replacement therapy is not without side-effects and it doesn't work for all women. The side-effects include persistent thrush infections, fluid retention, nausea and stomach upsets, migraine headaches, irritability, weight gain and breast soreness. One woman who reported 'acne, bad temper and change in nature' on oral oestrogens said she improved with transdermal oestrogen, which is transmitted through a patch on the skin.

Although the dose of hormones in HRT is lower than that in oral contraceptives, the side-effects are similar. If you have had trouble with the Pill, you are likely to experience difficulty with HRT. There is also a risk of gallstones, high blood pressure and thrombosis possibly leading to stroke, particularly where the oestrogen is given unopposed, that is, without progestin. There are different types of HRT, which use different oestrogens in varying dosages. If one combination doesn't work, another might. Women on hormones should stop smoking and keep their weight down.

Women taking HRT should expect that menopausal symptoms will recur when they stop taking the hormones. There is considerable debate among doctors about how long women should stay on it: some say they should stay on it for life, others say at least 15 years.

Women with menopausal symptoms might be helped by attending seminars on the subject held by the Family Planning Association. There are alternative treatments for menopausal symptoms, using drugs, herbs, vitamins, acupuncture, exercise and diet. Some helpful books on menopause are listed in the bibliography of this book.

Long-term risks and health care

The evidence about the long-term risks of hysterectomy is conflicting. Some studies have shown an increased risk of breast cancer; others show the risk actually decreases. It is not known whether hysterectomy with retention of the ovaries increases the risk of osteoporosis, which develops with oestrogen loss. When women take HRT in the appropriate dose the risk of osteoporosis is significantly decreased, although it is still not known what dose is the most effective in achieving this. A very small dose might prevent hot flushes, but not be much help in preventing osteoporosis. Risk factors for osteoporosis, beside oestrogen loss, are slight build, high alcohol consumption, smoking, lack of exercise and constant dieting. Overweight women, black women and Maori and Pacific Island women are at low risk of osteoporosis.

A recent study in the *New England Medical Journal* reported that having a hysterectomy doubles the risk of heart disease if both ovaries are removed, but that hormones can eliminate the additional risk. Women with one ovary intact had no additional risk. But once again the evidence so far is conflicting: other studies have shown increased risk. A similar pattern emerges with women taking oestrogen: some show more heart disease; some show less. There have been no completed studies so far on the effects of HRT (with progestin) on heart disease. If there is a beneficial effect of oestrogen, the progestin might cancel it out.

All women over 50 should have a mammogram or breast X-ray, to be repeated at three-yearly intervals or less, to monitor for breast changes that may mean cancer. This is not readily available in the public health system, but is available privately.

In the past it has been usual to say that women do not need smear tests after hysterectomy unless the operation was for cancer. It is now recommended that all women have regular smears after hysterectomy as carcinoma in situ can occur in the vagina. A vaginal vault smear every two or three years would be a good precaution.

Any woman on HRT should have regular check-ups for blood pressure, triglyceride levels (fatty substances in the blood) and cholesterol.

10

RECOVERY

Hysterectomy is major surgery and bodies take time to mend, so you will need to convalesce after getting home from hospital. Your family and friends should surround you with tender loving care and show their support in a practical way by taking over *all* the housework for the first few weeks. Don't do any jobs that involve stretching, bending or lifting, such as vacuuming and hanging out the washing. Someone will have to be available to help all day if you have pre-schoolers, as lifting them and taking care of them is out of the question. Fathers should take at least the first fortnight off work.

Don't expect to be able to do too much too soon. Take things slowly for the first three or four weeks and rest for part of each day. At first don't try to lift anything heavier than a jug of water. Activities can gradually be increased, and it is a good idea to also go for a walk and to try and increase the distance every day. A body will soon tire or ache if too much is expected of it, in which case it is important to slow down a little.

Try to avoid driving a car for the first month as, although it won't be physically harmful, you may well find that you are too tired and are unable to concentrate, particularly in heavy traffic. A sharp jolt if it is necessary to brake suddenly or a bumpy road can be painful.

It is important to know what is normal and what is not. While all women will have some vaginal bleeding when they first come home, and may need to use sanitary pads for several weeks, this should gradually taper off. Don't feel you are wasting your doctor's time by ringing back to report any worrying symptoms, for example, excessive bleeding, fever, unexpected pain or a smelly vaginal discharge. These may indicate infection or other problems that need further treatment. Complications can slow recovery. One woman in our survey wrote: 'I had fifteen months of treatment for a variety of complications before I began to feel well. None of these were mentioned to me before the operation, and I was made to feel guilty for not getting better.'

Most women, however, can expect an uneventful recovery. New Zealand doctors generally tell patients that they should be able to resume all their normal activities and go back to work after six weeks. This is probably over-optimistic for some women.

Margaret Ryan reported in an Australian survey that three-quarters of hysterectomy patients did not feel physically

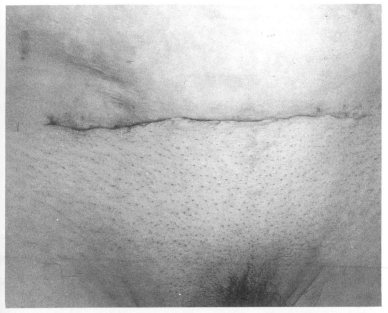

An abdominal hysterectomy incision, immediately after surgery.

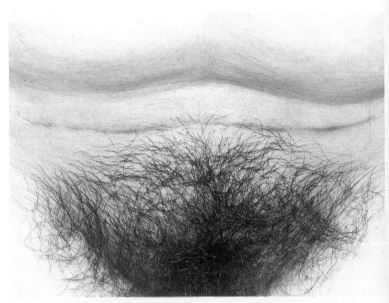

Six weeks after abdominal surgery the incision is healing well.

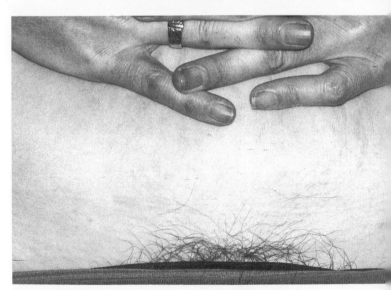

Two years after surgery, the scar is difficult to see.

recovered until 24 weeks after the operation, although by 6 weeks 70 percent were able to do any household work and by 8 weeks all those who had taken leave from work had returned.

In an English survey by C. Webb the average time before going back to work was even longer — 9.9 weeks. In this same survey it was noted that women who participated in energetic sports had resumed these by 4 months.

The rates quoted are average quotes. Individual recovery times vary considerably. In our survey some women were up and about milking the cows or tramping the hills within weeks of their hysterectomies but others said it took a year before they felt really fit again. Some women wrote that going back to work after six weeks was fine for them, but others felt very tired and stressed after a day's work at first. But once they had got over the initial tiredness they often felt an overwhelming sense of relief that the bad days were now behind them and that the quality of their lives had improved.

In our questionnaire we asked women how they felt about having a hysterectomy now. They could choose to write about anything they liked and some women wrote a good deal. Because women chose the most important things to mention, and missed other things out, some of our statistics don't tell the whole story. For example, 8 percent of women chose to mention problems in their sex life in answer to this question, whereas 22 percent had earlier ticked the box to say they had a less satisfactory sex life.

Overall 65 percent of the women expressed only positive feelings about having had their hysterectomy. When we added in the people with some mixed feelings (that is, they expressed both positive and negative feelings), a total of 81 percent of the women had something positive to say about their hysterectomy. They used words like 'terrific', 'thankful', 'no regrets', 'recommend one', 'liberated', 'satisfied', and 'glad'.

Twenty-seven percent of the women specifically mentioned an improvement in their health. They called themselves 'fit', 'active', 'well' and 'never better'. Some talked about self-image and said they felt 'younger', 'more feminine', 'cleaner', and 'more confident'.

> It was just a relief to be able to walk or run without the heavy dragging feeling I had, always continually carrying extra pads and tampons with me wherever I went. I had no depression, just relief.

> It felt so wonderful never to have to think about periods and contraception again.

> It was the best thing I ever did! I had not realised how much of my life was passing me by as I had been unable to go out to work. I now hold down a full-time job. Camping was something planned not to coincide with that time of the month. We can now go wherever we choose. I now play sport, something I had not done since the birth of my youngest son. Sex has improved, as I have more energy. I laugh and smile more than ever, and I wish I had done it earlier.

Our questionnaire showed that for 36 percent of women it was a totally positive experience. They felt positive beforehand, they had no complications and some time later they still felt only pleased about it.

On the other hand 10 percent of the women felt negative about everything. They had felt negative beforehand, they had complications and they still felt completely unhappy about it.

Overall 31 percent of women expressed some negative feelings about having had a hysterectomy. Fifteen percent had nothing but negative feelings now. About the same number — 14 percent — said they regretted having had the operation at all. These figures are alarmingly high and confirm our view that women need to be given much more information so that they make decisions that are right for them and that they feel happy about.

The words women used to describe these feelings were 'bitter', 'disappointed', 'depressed', 'sad', 'numb', 'can't accept it', and 'confused'.

Five percent of the women reported no improvement or a deterioration in their physical health. This was caused by complications, such as long-term bladder problems, or a lack of improvement in their original condition, while some women reported they had gained weight, felt 'fatigued', or became 'a nervous wreck'. Nine percent of women reported feeling negative about doctors and/or the hospital system. Eight percent mentioned negative effects on their sexuality (3 percent mentioned positive effects) and 4 percent were still unreconciled to their loss of fertility.

A few women felt they had aged, while others said they felt and looked younger. This is not really surprising if their health had been poor beforehand.

It is difficult to separate out the effects of hysterectomy from the normal ageing process. Hysterectomies are more frequently done on women over 40, when there is a tendency for the first grey hairs and wrinkles to appear, to have some facial hair growth and to put on weight. But some women were certain that their battle with middle age spread had started straight after the hysterectomy and blamed the operation.

One of the most interesting aspects of our survey was that we received so many replies from women who had had a hysterectomy a long time ago, sometimes several decades past. The general attitude was positive, although some women had continued to have health problems related to the hysterectomy. A small group of women had been unable to resolve their grief, and even after many years they felt upset, confused and not quite whole. It was noticeable that the women in the worst kind of turmoil felt that they had been very poorly informed about why their ovaries had been removed.

There were some uncertainties among the older women: confusion as to what would happen to them during the menopause, or feeling unsure whether menopause had already started. They had to guess from other symptoms such as hot flushes. But there were also some advantages.

I am pleased not to have menstrual and contraceptive problems that other women have as they get older. Tampax is so expensive!

For a few years I felt the occasional loss of fertility, especially as I had only one child. But now that I am getting past childbearing I feel very content and consider myself very lucky not to be having the numerous problems that my friends are having.

An unexpected spin-off was that women sometimes found an increased self-confidence after hysterectomy, and this could happen even if it had been a bad experience.

I guess in retrospect I have become stronger as a result and I am assertive now. I question professionals, and I ask for a second opinion, and I feel as if I have gone through the emotional part of the menopause, accepting the ageing, loss of childbearing potential. Now there is still the physical part of menopause to go but I feel strong, knowing I've come though it all so far.

Improved physical health had meant that women had been able to lead normal lives and had been able to hold down jobs and to look after their families. Some women had also felt confident to take on new challenges, a new career or a new leisure pursuit.

11

SEXUALITY

Sexual response after hysterectomy

Every woman will want to know if having a hysterectomy will affect her sexuality.

Sexuality is a vulnerable part of us involving all the complexities of self-expression, emotional satisfaction and well-being, intimacy, loving relationships, self-loving and sexual passion. But to quote Sheila Kitzinger, a common view of sex is 'what a man does to a woman on a Saturday night in bed . . . We have been conditioned by a society that sees the be-all and end-all of sex as intercourse and that devalues all the other aspects of female sexual experience.' Every woman is different and will have different concerns and needs. What our sexuality means to us reflects our age, culture, sexual orientation and preference, physical abilities, personal experience, ideals and values.

We often see our uterus as linked with our sexuality. It sheds its lining every month and is an outward sign of a woman's 'femaleness' and her ability to bear a child. Removing the uterus may seem a threat to a woman's sexual life and her view of herself as a complete woman.

Most early research on this subject was concerned primarily with how much sex women had after hysterectomy, rather than how good that sex was, and there was an emphasis on penis-in-vagina sex, to the exclusion of other kinds of sexual expression.

Recent research studies show that hysterectomy can significantly alter women's experience of sexual intercourse, but as in earlier research, the researchers didn't ask about masturbation or lesbian sex. The changes women experience are often just temporary, while the body adjusts to the effects of the surgery. Margaret Ryan's 1985 study of 90 Melbourne women found the majority reported an improved sexual life or no change following their hysterectomies. But a significant minority, just over one-quarter, reported an outcome unsatisfactory to them.

This Australian study and another study by Israeli researchers also showed that an unsatisfactory sexual outcome was linked with women not being given enough information about how a hysterectomy could affect them sexually. These findings highlight how important it is for women to make sure they have all the relevant information before they agree to this operation. It was apparent from our questionnaire that many women had been given little information before surgery. There might well have been fewer negative experiences if these women had been more fully informed.

Women answering our questionnaire had a range of sexual responses after hysterectomy, from those who felt ecstatic to women who were in deep despair because their enjoyment of sex seemed to have disappeared altogether. Nearly half the women in our survey did not tick boxes for either improved sex life or diminished sex life; presumably for them sex remained much the same. Increased sexual pleasure was reported by 32 percent of the women, but 22 percent were unsatisfied with their sex lives after their hysterectomies. The women could tick boxes for 'less satisfactory sex life' and 'difficulty reaching orgasm'. Eleven percent ticked both boxes, and 14 percent reported having difficulty reaching orgasm.

It is interesting to note that our rate of 22 percent of women with less satisfactory sex lives closely matches Margaret Ryan's rate in her study. The scientific quibbles that could be raised about the way we did our survey are not applicable to her research. We asked women to reply in retrospect and there could have been an element of bias in who chose to fill the questionnaire out and who didn't. Critics could argue that 'dissatisfied' women might be more highly motivated to take part in the survey. Margaret Ryan's was a prospective study: she talked to the women before the hysterectomy and followed them through, interviewing them at intervals afterwards. Yet her results are much the same as ours, reinforcing our view that we heard from a good cross-section of women.

For the women in our survey who said their sexual pleasure had increased the change for the better could be dramatic. Before surgery they had felt run down and irritable. The removal of the uterus meant they were now rid of uncomfortable and distressing symptoms, for example, heavy bleeding and painful periods, and returned to good health and an improved sex life. One of the respondents wrote that she felt 'all woman, my hysterectomy has allowed me to enjoy my sexuality and femininity to a much greater extent than before'. Another woman saw her hysterectomy as a turning point in her life:

> I feel better than I have felt for 10 years. I really hadn't realised how my life was totally dominated by a small internal organ. I don't miss it at all and I certainly don't feel any less female. I am now clean and sweet smelling at all times and have a great deal of energy. My sex life is really great and I feel a complete woman in all facets of my life.

Some women found that orgasm after their hysterectomies was a sharper and more intense sensation. One woman said she became orgasmic after 20 years of non-orgasmic marriage. Another woman, detailing the positive effects of hysterectomy on her personal life, commented: 'My husband loves me as intensely as always and I have to tell you that he gave me an oral orgasm 10 days after the hysterectomy to my great delight and pleasure.'

It was not just the return to good health that allowed women to enjoy their sexuality more, but often also the psychological benefits of not having periods and not being able to get pregnant again. 'My sex life improved out of sight — no more worry each month re pregnancy.'

For some women who had previously not been sexual while they were menstruating, there was also the delight in being able to have sex every day of the month. 'I must say I like always being available for sex at any time now that I don't have periods.'

Coping with difficulties

Women are generally advised after having a hysterectomy to wait until after their six-weekly check-up before having an orgasm or vaginal penetration as part of sex. An orgasm may be painful as the muscle contractions pull on healing tissue. This wait will give the wound at the top of the vaginal vault where the cervix used to be time to heal properly. The expectation is that after this time women will go home and resume their sex life as before. But life isn't always that straightforward. A British survey of 69 women found 41 had initial difficulties with sex. These included difficulty with penetration, a dry vagina, pain during penetrative sex, lack of sexual desire and bleeding. After a few months, however, the majority of women reported enjoying sex more than before surgery and felt like being sexual more often.

Difficulty with penetration and pain during intercourse may be due to scar tissue, shortening and tightening of the vagina, or temporary shrinkage (called post-operative contracture). Also a woman's vagina usually expands and balloons upwards during sexual arousal and this may not occur to the same extent after a hysterectomy.

Stopping having sex is not the answer, as the tissues need to be stretched and lubricated. It is usually okay to have sex if you can flex the muscles in your abdomen, tighten the muscles around your vagina and grip hard without causing pain. Doing exercises to strengthen these muscles will help. Kegel's exercise is described in chapter 4.

If we have been with the same partner a long time, sometimes we don't spend enough time with some of the lovely intimate sexual things two people can do together, such as kissing, touching, even talking about things we like about the other person and the things we want to do to or with them. When you make love, delay penetration until you are very aroused and make sure your partner is very gentle. Having an orgasm before penetration is almost guaranteed to ensure that your vagina will be at its most receptive and reduce the possibility of tension and pain. Your lover putting his or her mouth on you or touching you is a way of making you aroused and wet before a penis or fingers go into your vagina. If you are not used to oral sex, this idea may be a bit startling, but once you have got over being shy or embarrassed, you may find whole new possibilities have opened up to you.

A dry vagina can be moistened with a water-soluble lubricant, such as K-Y jelly. Lubricants can be bought from your local supermarket or chemist.

It helps to talk to your partner if you are having problems, so that the two of you can co-operate and make love in a way that doesn't hurt you. If you find it a hard subject to bring up, maybe you could start by showing your lover this section of the book.

If you continue to have difficulty, talk to your doctor. She or he may need to stretch your vagina if it is too tight, or cauterise (seal with heat) blood vessels that are still bleeding. One woman described this process: 'The corrective surgery after the hysterectomy was the cauterising of a tiny spot that hadn't healed. This was causing sharp pains during intercourse. Since that was done I have never felt better.'

Fourteen percent of the women in our survey said they had difficulty reaching orgasm. Although doctors have been inclined to tell women it was their fault because they didn't relax enough, or they were imagining it, research indicates that this is not so.

Masters and Johnson, who have researched women's responses during sexual activity, found that the pelvic area, including the uterus, becomes congested with blood before orgasm. This congestion may cause the feelings of arousal. When women reach orgasm, the uterus and pelvic area rhythmically contracts, helping release the congestion. So when the uterus is removed orgasm can feel less intense and may be shorter. Most women feel the centre of their orgasms in their clitoris, but those who feel them deeper inside might notice a difference in intensity. Some women also enjoy the sensation of a penis or fingers pushing up against the cervix during deep penetration. Once the cervix has gone that's gone too.

For some women these are negative changes, but they need to be balanced against the positive aspects of having a hysterectomy. Women can compensate for these changes by experimenting with different ways of making love. One woman wrote: 'I've wondered why the cramps I used to get after we'd made love disappeared. Now I know why. It takes a lot more stimulation before orgasm happens, but it is still enjoyable.' For others the loss of intensity of their orgasms made them regret their hysterectomy.

Women sometimes feel pressured to have orgasms during sex, and if they don't, they can feel they have failed. Shere Hite and other researchers have suggested that 70 percent of women don't reach orgasm solely from penetrative intercourse with a male partner. A more women-oriented definition of sex would include massage, whole body touching, focus on the clitoris as well as the vagina and enjoying our partner's fingers and tongue. Sex viewed this way can be enjoyable for women whether or not we reach orgasm.

Very occasionally women completely lose their sexual arousal and interest. This was particularly distressing for one woman. 'The doctor said, of course I could still have a sex life. He never mentioned I may not want one. I still feel like physical contact and use some lubrication. This helps prevent vaginal discomfort. But nowadays it is a companiable exercise with my husband.'

This loss of sexual interest and arousal may be related to changes in the balance of hormones in the body. This is discussed in chapter 9.

Even when women feel their sex lives have suffered, they can improve over time. 'On the sexual side I felt dead inside for quite a while, but now that I have recovered from the tiredness this area is as good as it ever was.' Another woman experienced 'ups and downs sexually' and expressed hope that 'it's settling down as my system settles down'. She went on to speculate that 'it seems a possibility that not a lot can be done to circumvent the whole sense of loss, mood swings and grief'. Adequate information and counselling before and after the operation may have helped. In our survey lesbians did not identify themselves, but they share some of these feelings and difficulties. It can take time to sort it all out.

Some partners were also affected by a hysterectomy. Men were sometimes too scared to have penetrative sex with their partners in case it hurt them. Some men treated their partners as if they weren't capable of sex any more. Sometimes they were scared that they might catch something, especially cancer. This can't happen. Not being able to have children with their partner also grieved some men.

A hysterectomy in itself cannot cause or solve problems you may already have with your sexuality, sexual relationships or sexual response. This may be a time to re-evaluate your feelings and seek help. We have listed some helpful books in the bibliography. Counselling services can also be useful.

As Sheila Kitzinger notes, sexuality is more than what we manage to achieve in bed, it 'consists of a whole range of experiences that are not just genital. Sex involves the whole body and is expressed in different ways at different times in a woman's life'. Sexuality infuses the whole of life.

12

DEPRESSION AND GRIEF

Depression

Nearly 70 percent of the women in our survey reported that they had had no feelings of depression after their hysterectomy. In fact many said they had had only positive thoughts afterwards and some attributed it to their own positive mental attitude.

Thirty-one percent of the women in our survey reported that they had been depressed after their hysterectomy. In chapter 9 we discussed one possible cause, loss of ovarian function, but there are other possible causes.

Mood swings, feeling down and being easily upset are quite normal after a hysterectomy. The body has had a major shock and the anaesthetic can in itself depress — the whole experience can be quite traumatic and will take time to get over. Having this reaction does not mean there will be ongoing depression or that a deeper depression will develop.

Hysterectomy is a stressful event, so it is useful to know about stress, how to recognise the warning signs and how to cope with it. The physical warning signs include: headaches, problems with sleeping, tiredness and lethargy, palpitations, heavy sweating, tight and painful muscles, constipation, indigestion, loss of sexual desire and high blood pressure.

The mental warning signs include: inability to relax, poor concentration and memory, difficulty in finishing tasks, irritability, impulsive behaviour and depressed moods.

Women who took part in our survey had often had one of these symptoms after their hysterectomy. We didn't ask in the questionnaire how long the negative effects lasted and it was clear that depression meant different things to different people. Sometimes it was only transitory and was finished by the time they left hospital. For other women it lasted much longer.

> I am still [a year later] pleased to be rid of the physical problems, but there have been obvious emotional side-effects for which I was totally unprepared. Since the operation we have moved to another city. I have suffered violent mood swings and depression. Instead of the calm, confident professional woman I was, I am now very much lacking in confidence and easily upset. I have become very selfish and try to protect myself from too much contact with the outside world. As a result of reading your article I have come to understand that this personality change is not just my not adapting well to the environment, but the result of having a hysterectomy. I have visited my GP and outlined my symptoms. He tells me that I might be reading to him a textbook of problems associated with hysterectomy and that this operation is the one most commonly associated with depression.

Australian researcher Margaret Ryan has studied and written about the problem of depression after hysterectomy. She has summarised a number of risk factors identified by various researchers that may mean some women are more predisposed than others to becoming depressed after a hysterectomy.

Women under 40 years of age and women who have not completed their families are more likely to become depressed. It is not the number of children a woman has, but whether she wanted to have more that is the key factor. Divorced and separated women are prone to depression because they may lack support. Women whose husbands are unhelpful suffer in the same way.

Not having a job outside the home is a risk factor, whereas being employed protects against depression as it gives women additional opportunities for social support and self-esteem.

Women who have psychological problems at the time of the hysterectomy or who have had them in the past are more likely to get depressed, as are women who find stress hard to handle. Women whose lives centre on reproduction and motherhood can feel depressed because losing their ability to have children may damage their self-esteem, even if they didn't plan to have any more children.

Other stressful events occurring at the same time as the hysterectomy, such as the death of a friend, losing a job, or a teenage child leaving home can trigger depression. In our survey, one woman who described herself as 'by nature a fairly positive person' and 'always on the go' outlined the severe depression she had experienced in the year after her hysterectomy. In that time she had also had 'our daughter's marriage break up, almost lost a wee granddaughter through illness, my husband got cancer and we had to go to Wellington for a month'. She spent some time in a psychiatric hospital and was still seeing a psychiatrist when she wrote.

It has been common in the past to explain some post-hysterectomy depression as really being about women ageing. Most women who have hysterectomies are in their forties. They are approaching menopause, their children may be leaving home and their parents may need extra care. As women get older they may feel less attractive in our youth-oriented society. One of our respondents (41 years old, two children) expressed some of these concerns.

> I'm glad to be rid of the continual pain and bleeding, but am experiencing difficulty in coming to terms with the fact that as far as reproducing goes I am useless. This tends to affect other aspects of my married life. I don't know if it is altogether the hysterectomy that has caused this, but also the fact that my children are independent now and don't really need me. This all adds up to a feeling of being useless after twenty years of being a wife and mother. I have had a part-time job for years, but now find that I am not trained for anything positive. I have gone back

to night school to do fifth form accounting, so this may lead to something.

As more women have fulfilling careers and can look forward to successes in their forties and fifties, depression from such causes must diminish, as we suspect it has begun to already.

It is important to remember that although researchers have identified these 'risk factors', depression is by no means inevitable even if you have them. Many women do not experience depression at all. And women who feel down for a few weeks should not be too concerned. A normal depression will soon pass, but a serious depression refuses to lift. It is important to be able to recognise serious depression and do something about it. Such a depression, if left unattended to, can get worse and seriously affect physical and mental health.

The Canadian Mental Health Association has reported that signs of the kind of depression that may require professional help include:

- A specific mood change of long duration: sadness, loneliness, apathy, fatigue
- Negative ideas about oneself that don't conform to reality
- Unrealistic assumptions of self-blame
- Marked changes in a person's physiology such as extreme weight loss or gain.

Stress management
Women can often take some steps of their own to rid themselves of stress and depression. The New Zealand Mental Health Foundation has suggested a six-point management plan.

1. Eat a properly balanced diet.
2. Take regular physical exercise.
3. Use relaxation techniques.
4. Plan your time — make lists of things to do but avoid

setting goals because if you fail to achieve them you will face more stress.

5. Relax — don't build catastrophes out of minor nuisances.
6. Share your worries with friends or relatives. If you are under a lot of strain, talk to your doctor or call a telephone counsellor.

Women who like company will almost certainly be able to find a group to join. There are groups on relaxation, assertiveness training and coping skills available in most communities and if they are run by community organisations they usually don't cost much. There are plenty of opportunities for exercise too. In some cities the YMCA runs Y's Walking, which is particularly recommended because it is not too strenuous but still allows a reasonable fitness level to be achieved.

Reducing depression

It is very important to acknowledge that you are depressed and to tell someone. Having a sympathetic friend can be as effective as going to a professional counsellor. Reading about the experiences other women have had and how they coped can help you to recognise that what you are experiencing is not unique and provide you with some useful coping strategies.

If you are depressed it is especially important to look after yourself, and to take time out for your own needs — eat well, keep fit and do relaxation exercises.

Try to work out why you are depressed. If you feel it is because of losing your womb keep reminding yourself that you are still a unique and special person and that your femininity does not depend on having a womb.

It can feel particularly painful if people are unkind or unhelpful after a hysterectomy. This can be a symptom that there is something wrong with the relationship and this may need working out.

A challenge such as a new job that may now be in reach because of improved physical health can help to fend off depression. You may feel that you can't face a major change right away, but you should make every effort not to stay in a rut but to keep moving ahead and making new decisions, however little — picking up the phone and talking to an old friend, getting dressed and going somewhere for a walk, joining a night class may not seem like much but it can all help. Don't, however, set yourself unrealistic goals.

Try not to give up hope. Remember that all depressions lift eventually. Positive thinking is very good too. Let your imagination work for you — imagine yourself as successful, interesting, doing new things rather than failing or feeling neglected.

But if your depression doesn't go away, don't leave it too long — you don't have to wait until it gets really bad before seeking professional help. Don't be embarrassed about it. Depression is very common and it can happen to anybody.

If you have come to the point where you need professional help it is not a bad idea to start with your GP. A doctor can rule out or treat any physical health problems that could be causing mood problems. But beware of using doctors as counsellors for emotional problems — many lack skills and most have little training in this area. Although some women have found their doctors to be very helpful and to be good listeners, others have had very poor advice.

Doctors should be able to tell women about the range of counselling services available to them in the community. It is also possible to get this information from the Citizens' Advice Bureau.

There is a wide range of professionals who can offer help. There are two kinds of university trained professionals — psychiatrists (medical doctors with specialised training in mental health) and psychologists (graduates in psychology, the science of human behaviour). Many other counsellors have been trained in a variety of schemes, and if they have reached an acceptable level they can become members of the New Zealand Association of Psychotherapists and Counsellors. It is probably wise to go to someone with this kind of professional experience, although an unqualified person can sometimes also have good counselling skills. You should always find out beforehand what their qualifications are, what sorts of experience they have and what kinds of therapy they have to offer.

Like many other emotional problems, there is no one specific cure for depression. Each individual requires different types of therapy or treatment, so it is very important to find a therapist whose therapies and personality suit your needs.

In her book *Mental Health for Women* Hilary Haines has pointed out that there are many instances of therapists being harmful to women by attempting to make them conform, or adjust to their prescribed roles. If, for example, a therapist holds the view that all every woman really wants is a man and babies and that their work ambitions are neurotic, it can be very damaging to a woman who cannot have any more children. If a therapist has sexist attitudes, is not helping with your problems, or you simply don't get on well, it is best not to persevere but to find someone else.

How much the therapist charges will also need to be taken into account. Some Area Health Boards have community mental health centres whose trained staff can provide a free service. An example is the Auburn Centre on the North Shore in Auckland, where there is always a woman therapist available to work with female patients. You do not need to go to your doctor first to have access to this type of service — you can refer yourself. There are also services, such as Presbyterian Support, that are fairly affordable. If you have no medical insurance, or if medical insurance doesn't cover all consultations, going to a therapist privately can be very expensive. Find out how much it will cost before you go.

If you do not like taking pills you may wish to avoid a doctor or a psychiatrist and go instead to psychologist or counsellor who may be able to achieve the same results without drugs. However, the drugs doctors and psychiatrists may prescribe can be very useful in the short run.

Drugs should always only be a temporary measure to help control the symptoms. When the symptoms are under control, the therapist should then help the woman to see why she feels the way she does. The professional should also try to help the woman understand how depression can happen and how to avoid it happening again.

Depression after a hysterectomy is often, but not always, linked to grief. There may be physical problems or other problems related to sexuality or to the relationship with a partner. As depression after hysterectomy is so commonly linked to grief, however, it is important to find out about grief and what to do about it.

Grief

It is perfectly normal to grieve about losing a womb. This is a healthy reaction to a significant loss. It may be painful, but it can't be avoided. If emotions are not allowed to come to the surface, they can't be dealt with and healing can't take place.

When a hysterectomy is first suggested to a woman she may feel shocked, panic-stricken, depressed, guilty or angry. By recognising that these feelings are related to grief, allowing them to come to the surface and facing them, women are able to start working through their grief. Grief can be anticipated, and much of the process can be worked through before a hysterectomy; this is another good reason why women should not allow themselves to be rushed into surgery.

Grief often follows a pattern, and there are usually five stages: denial, rage and anger, bargaining, depression, and acceptance. Not everyone will experience all of these emotions or experience them in this sequence. People can also have many of these feelings simultaneously, but one feeling usually dominates and this feeling will determine behaviour at a particular time.

It is important to identify exactly what you feel you are losing and only you can identify how significant that loss is. Recent research suggests that it is quite common nowadays for women not to feel any great sense of loss about their hysterectomy, and there were many women in our questionnaire who bore this out. The reason fewer women today feel a great sense of loss may be the changing role of women. There has in recent years been less emphasis on the importance of reproduction for women's self-esteem. Women are also much more knowledgeable about what the surgery involves and how it affects their bodies, and they are able to participate more actively in the decision. Some women, however, experience a tremendous upsurge of painful emotions after hysterectomy, and the significance of the loss for that person determines the depth of the response.

It can be difficult for women today to identify exactly why they are grieving. We have been brought up in a society that has given us mixed messages. On the one hand there is the feeling that girls can do anything, and on the other hand there is still a widely held belief that what women really want to do most, and do best, is have babies and nurture them. Little girls get the dolls and little boys the cars.

With all this confusion about whether a woman's self-esteem is derived from the fulfilment of biological function, it is no wonder that women often feel a range of conflicting emotions and that it is sometimes difficult for them to say exactly how they feel.

Some women do most of their grieving before surgery, others do it afterwards. Many women feel tearful in hospital on the third day after surgery. Knowing what they are grieving for and seeing what this part of their bodies looks like can help some women. In some hospitals a photograph is taken of the womb after it is removed. In this way it gives the woman something tangible over which to grieve.

It is difficult to say whether the tiredness, irritability and emotional ups and downs that many women experience when they go home are related to grief or are after-effects of the surgery itself. Grief can cause physical symptoms, such as changes in bowel habits, headaches, stomach aches and insomnia.

A career woman or someone who has already completed her family can still feel an acute sense of loss, while some women can be surprisingly accepting of their situation. This is because some women are more susceptible to grief and less able to resolve it.

There is a recurring theme in the literature about hysterectomy that women who have not coped well with losses previously or who have suffered from depression beforehand are particularly at risk and are less likely to make a good recovery. In such studies it is usually the woman's individual make-up and coping strategies that are seen as determining how well she is able to resolve her grief. But the people around her can also help or hinder her.

Women who are vulnerable can be helped to cope by people around them — partners have a very important role to play and it is essential that they understand exactly what is happening and show that they care. If family and friends are aware of what a uterus is and what it can mean, it can make a lot of difference to the woman. If the people around her are not supportive, if there are other crises in her life, or if she is too busy looking after her children to take time out for herself, a reaction may set in later.

> For three to six months it was marvellous to feel so well without all the prolapse. I had a two-and-a-half-year-old and a ten-month-old. From six months I coped with feeling very inadequate as a woman. Friends were all having babies, and I couldn't. The right of choice had gone. It took 18 months before I began to feel pleased that I had had it.

Some women are unable to resolve their grief by themslves. A small group of women who replied to our questionnaire were in this position. Years after the event they still felt confused, upset and not quite whole.

The sensible part of my brain understands that I was never allowed a grief or bereavement time. It was always 'The operation is over, you're well now.' I was back rushing round for other people within three weeks, smiling, working, saying I was fine — but I wasn't. I felt then, and I still do, as if part of me died. There has never been someone to tell this to until now.

Women who feel like this can be helped if they go to a counsellor who is skilled in the area of grief. You can contact a grief counsellor through your GP or you can go directly to an Area Health Board community health centre — these provide a free service. A counsellor will help you to reconstruct the past and allow you to work through all the distressing and painful feelings which you are not able to work through on your own. By doing this you will eventually be able to remember it without distress.

It isn't possible to say how long it will take to resolve the grief about a hysterectomy. Women who really don't mind losing their womb can get quite annoyed if people think they must be feeling sad. But for women who did feel it was a significant part of their body it could take more than a year. Sometimes when someone thinks they have finished with grief it can reappear briefly, years later, triggered off by an object, an anniversary or a person connected with the event.

For those women who find it a painful experience there can be a spin-off. Some women in our survey said that they had emerged stronger for the experience, and they felt that their confidence in themselves and their ability to cope had increased.

13

NETWORKING

At the back of overseas books about hysterectomy there is usually a comprehensive list of support groups for women to contact if they want further help and information. Unfortunately we are unable to provide such a list. Although self-help groups are also a feature of the New Zealand way of life, very few groups have been set up especially for hysterectomy patients. Some of the women who answered our questionnaire said they would have liked information and support from other women who had had a hysterectomy, or they would have liked to help other women in the same situation.

It is not difficult to start a self-help group, but it is important to gather information about how such a group is usually organised. You need to know how to plan and organise a meeting, and to think about the aims and structure of the group. A decision will also have to be made as to whether to ask a health professional to help. Having such a person present at the meetings may create difficulties for women whose experiences with the medical profession have been distressing. It may be more appropriate to invite a nurse or social worker to be available as an adviser or consultant to the group, rather than being a member who attends meetings. It is also necessary to work out how any costs incurred in publicity or educational material can be recouped.

The Mental Health Foundation in Auckland has published a small manual called *Getting Started*, which gives comprehensive, practical advice on how to set up a self-help group. It can be obtained from the Mental Health Foundation (272 Parnell Road, Auckland).

There may be people in the community who would be able to assist in setting up a self-help group. It is worth contacting the local women's health centre, the social work department of a hospital, a community mental health centre or a Citizens' Advice Bureau to ask if anyone is available to help, or whether they have a room or other resources that can be used free of charge.

One organisation that specialises in providing resources for self-help groups is the North Shore Community Health Network, which operates from Raeburn House in Milford, Auckland. This is a voluntary community-based organisation whose focus is to enable people to achieve good health. They provide information to North Shore women on how to set up groups and will give ongoing help and support.

Once the groundwork has been done other women can be invited to join the group. Contact can be made through suburban newspapers, word of mouth, women's health centres, local hospitals or doctors' practices.

Sometimes local self-help groups are part of a national organisation. An example of how a support network can be organised on a national scale is the VZB (Women without a Womb) in the Netherlands. VZB grew out of a series of menopause sessions run by VIDO, a Dutch organisation for menopausal women. Many of the hysterectomy patients who attended had horrifying stories to tell about doctors' attitudes, their treatment and unexpected after-effects. These women decided to start a separate national self-help network with two aims: to support women both before and after hysterectomy and to lobby the medical profession so that they would provide women with better information and more adequate and sensitive treatment.

The VZB has a nation-wide telephone service. It collects and disseminates literature about hysterectomy. It encourages women to set up self-help groups in their local communities and provides training sessions for group facilitators. It organises lectures and provides the media with information about hysterectomy. The VZB also writes its own information pamphlets and monitors the pamphlets given to women in hospitals.

Unlike Dutch women, New Zealand women often have to fossick around for what they need and depend on the medical profession for advice. Having to search for information and help is an additional stress, especially for women who are not feeling well or are upset about the operation.

Although hysterectomy support groups are few and far between, there are other avenues of help worth trying. In some areas there are women's health centres, such as Fertility Action in Auckland, or The Health Alternatives for Women in Christchurch, where there is an information file with articles about hysterectomy from a feminist perspective. Women's health centres often have a 'hot and cold' file about local doctors, so that women can find out which doctor is likely to be sympathetic. Women also find a sympathetic ear at their local Family Planning Association clinic, some of which run menopause support sessions. Women who have specific complaints about their treatment can contact a group, such as the Christchurch Patient's Rights group, which may be able to act as an advocate for them. The patient advocates who will soon be appointed in public hospitals will have an important role to play in protecting the rights of patients.

Hysterectomy patients' interests would be much better served if there was an organisation set up especially for them. We very much hope that in the not too distant future some New Zealand women might follow the lead of other countries and start the ball rolling.

THE HYSTERECTOMY SURVEY

Lynne S. Giddings   Pamela J. Wood

A questionnaire on hysterectomy was published in the *New Zealand Woman's Weekly* in April 1987.

In an article by Sandra Coney, 'Do you *really* have to have a hysterectomy?', Lyn Potter requested *NZWW* readers to complete and return the questionnaire so that a fuller picture of women's experience of hysterectomy could be obtained. The response was quite overwhelming. Women from all over New Zealand, 987 in total, returned the questionnaire. Many wrote accompanying letters, some pages long, detailing their experiences. It became evident that for many women, having a hysterectomy had been a significant event in their lives, whether the experience had been positive or negative.

The limitation of this survey is that it was restricted to *NZWW* readers who chose to respond. The results of the study, therefore, are not representative of all New Zealand women who have had a hysterectomy. It also should be noted that the range of information that could be obtained by the survey was restricted because of the requirements of the *NZWW* to limit the questionnaire to one page. It is important, however, that the experiences of these 987 women be acknowledged and recorded. A copy of the questionnaire is included at the end of this appendix.

Profile of respondents

Age

The total number of women who responded to the questionnaire (respondents) was 987. Their ages ranged from 25 to 84 years. The majority of women (738 women; 74 percent of total) were aged between 35 and 54 with the largest age group 40 to 44 (213 women; 22 percent of total). Thirteen women were 29 years and under and 40 (1.82 percent) 65 years and over.

Number of children

The majority of women reported having two or three children. It was not clear, however, whether these were children all born before the hysterectomy or whether new household arrangements, for example, adoption and stepchildren, affected family numbers.

Ethnic groups

The majority of respondents (951; 96 percent of total) described their ethnicity as Pakeha (European). When we compare the reported ethnicity of respondents in this study with the ethnic profile of *NZWW* readers, we can see that Maori, Pacific Island

Figure 1: Comparison of reported ethnicity of respondents with the ethnic profile of NZWW readers

	Pakeha (European)	Maori	Pacific Islander	Other
Survey (N = 987)	96.35% (951)	1.51% (15)	0.2% (2)	0.19% (19)
NZWW* (N=899 000)	87.43% (786 000)	7.29% (70 000)	3.23% (29 000)	1.56% (14 000)

* Source: AGB: Media 1988 Magazine Survey No. 2.

nationals and other ethnic groups are markedly under-represented (see fig. 1). There could be a number of possible reasons for this. Fewer Maori and Pacific Island women have hysterectomies; and a questionnaire is not always the most culturally appropriate way of finding out information of a personal nature.

Timing of hysterectomy

As might be expected, the largest single group of women (29 percent) reported having had their hysterectomy in the previous two years, that is, 1985, 1986 and early 1987. An equal number of women, however, had their hysterectomies before this, with a few in the 1950s and 1960s. Four women reported having had the operation in the 1940s, and filling in the questionnaire after this length of time could be an indication of the significance of the experience to them.

Figure 2: Age of respondents at time of hysterectomy

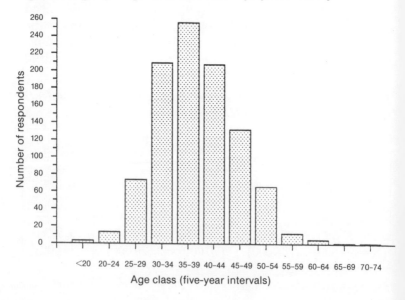

Age of respondents at time of hysterectomy

Figure 2 sets out in five-year intervals the age of respondents at the time they had the hysterectomy. The largest group was aged between 35 and 39 years. Three women were 19 years old at the time of hysterectomy. One had the operation because of infection, the second for endometriosis and the third at the time of giving birth by Caesarian section.

Results of the survey

Reasons for the hysterectomy

The question 'Why did you have a hysterectomy?' gave respondents a check-list of 10 reasons that might have applied to

Figure 3: Reasons for hysterectomy

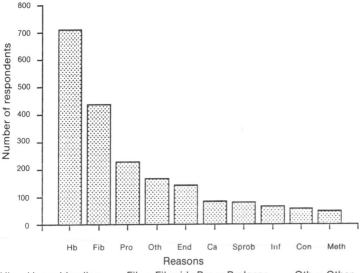

Hb = Heavy bleeding   Fib = Fibroids Pro = Prolapse   Oth = Other
End = Endometriosis   Ca = Cancer   Sprob = Problems after sterilisation
Inf = Infection   Con = Problems after contraception
Meth = Method of sterilisation

their situation. They could check more than one reason and most women did. Figure 3 sets out in graph form the main reasons they gave. Heavy bleeding was the most common reason (709 women or 72 percent) and was combined with the next most frequently stated reason, fibroids, in 326 cases.

What was removed
The majority of women, 70 percent, reported that the uterus alone was removed, 12 percent that one ovary was removed and 12 percent that both ovaries had been removed at the time of operation. A total of 50 respondents (5 percent) were not sure what specifically had been removed during the surgery.

Adequacy of information (informed consent)
In reply to the question, 'Did you feel you were given enough information to agree to the operation?', 676 women (68 percent) stated 'yes', and 311 (32 percent) 'no'. We do not know, however, what information was given except in relation to possible negative effects of the hysterectomy (see below).

Information concerning negative effects of hysterectomy
Respondents were asked if their doctor had informed them of any possible negative effects of the hysterectomy. A total of 667 women (68 percent) ticked 'no' and 320 (32 percent) ticked 'yes'. Figure 4 sets out in order of stated frequency the most commonly given possible negative effects. To this question respondents could tick more than one effect. Of the 320 women who had been given information about possible negative effects, 178 (56 percent) indicated that they had been informed that they might get depressed after surgery.

The analysis of the results of the questionnaire revealed that it would have been useful and interesting to include a question concerning the information given to the women about possible positive effects following a hysterectomy.

Figure 4: Information given about possible negative effects following hysterectomy

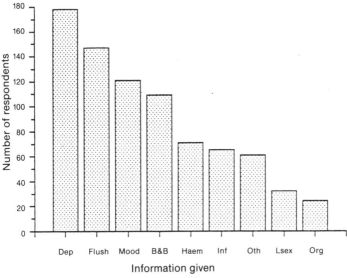

Dep = Depression   Flush = Hot flushes   B&B = Bladder & bowel
Haem = Haemorrhage   Mood = Mood swings   Oth = Other
Lsex = Less satisfactory sex life   Inf = Infection
Org = Difficulty reaching orgasm

Negative effects experienced following hysterectomy

Figure 5 sets out the actual negative effects the respondents reported experiencing following their hysterectomies. Altogether 636 women (64 percent) reported having one or more negative effects. They could tick more than one effect. With the exception of depression and hot flushes, the order of frequency is different from the possible negative effects their doctors told them about.

Figure 6 indicates the relationship between information given by the doctors about possible negative effects and negative effects actually experienced by the women. Respondents who were not

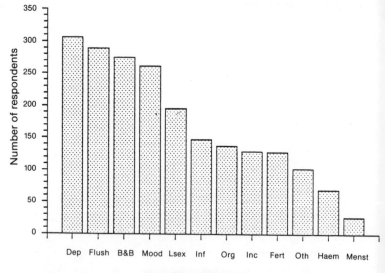

Figure 5: Negative effects experienced following hysterectomy

Number of respondents (y-axis, 0 to 350)

Negative effects (x-axis): Dep, Flush, B&B, Mood, Lsex, Inf, Org, Inc, Fert, Oth, Haem, Menst

Dep = Depression   Flush = Hot flushes   Mood = Mood swings
Lsex = Less satisfactory sex life   Inf = Infection   Oth = Other
Org = Difficulty reaching orgasm   Inc = Feeling incomplete as a woman
B&B = Bladder & bowel   Haem = Haemorrhage
Menst = Regret at loss of menstruation   Fert = Grief at loss of fertility

given any information reported experiencing more negative effects following their hysterectomies than the better informed women. The exception was women who had been told of the possible complication of haemorrhage and had then experienced it. These results suggest, therefore, that providing information about possible negative effects does not necessarily encourage women to experience them.

We also looked at whether women who experienced negative effects received treatment and found that, overall, few women were given treatment. The group which most frequently received treatment was women with infections — 64 percent of these women received help. Around a third of women who had depression, hot flushes and bowel and bladder problems were treated. Of note is the lack of treatment and/or counselling for negative effects in the area of sexuality. Only 1 percent of women who had problems with orgasm and 2 percent of women with a less satisfactory sex life received any help.

Figure 6: The relationship between information given and experience of negative effects

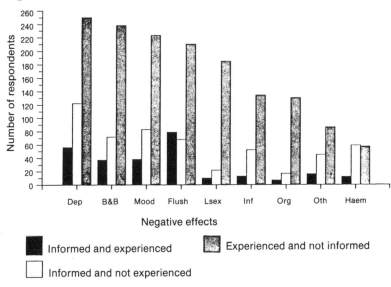

Positive effects experienced following hysterectomy

In total 938 (95 percent) of the 987 respondents reported having experienced one or more positive effects following their hysterectomies. Respondents could tick more than one effect.

Figure 7 sets out the positive effects the women reported experiencing. 'Relief of symptoms' was ticked by 828 women (84 percent), and 816 (83 percent) ticked 'freedom from periods'. It is interesting to note that the three physical positive effects were reported by more women than the psycho-sexual positive effects.

155

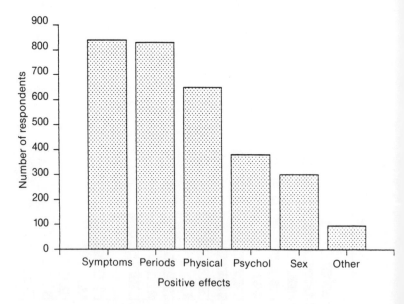

Symptoms = Relief of symptoms   Periods = Freedom from periods
Physical = Improved physical health   Psychol = Improved psychological
health   Sex = Increased sexual pleasure.

A comparison of the respondents who experienced negative and/or positive effects gave the following results: 594 women (60 percent) experienced both positive and negative effects; 344 (35 percent) positive effects only; 42 (4 percent) negative effects only; and 7 women experienced neither.

Figure 8 gives an indication of the relationship of informed consent with the women's experiences of positive and negative effects. From this graph it can be seen that the majority of women who reported having experienced only positive effects reported that they received adequate information prior to their operations. Conversely, the majority of women who reported having experienced only negative effects, reported they had *not* received adequate information prior to their operations.

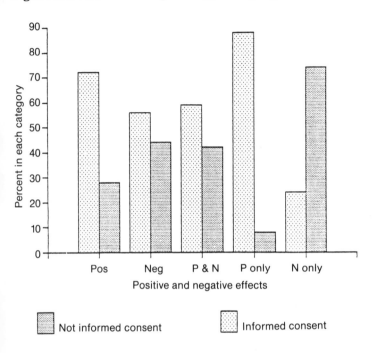

Figure 8: Positive and negative effects by informed consent

Legend: Not informed consent; Informed consent

Outcome

Question 12 of the survey asked respondents to recall and describe their feelings at the time they had their hysterectomies. Question 13 asked how they were feeling, at the time of filling out the questionnaire, about having had their hysterectomies. When analysed, key words from both questions fitted into the seven main categories listed here.

1. Health and general condition.
2. Health care system.
3. Support systems.
4. Feelings about the operation.
5. Self-image.

6. Personal relationships and sexuality.
7. Fertility.

Words written by the respondents were assigned within each category according to whether they conveyed a positive or negative meaning; for example, 'rushed' or 'unprepared' were listed as negative and 'vital' as positive. It is important to note that respondents were not asked specific questions about these categories, they were asked to comment on their feelings. The words used, therefore, reflect the significance of their experience to them, as they chose what they commented on. The results have been summarised in Figure 9.

It is anticipated that more detailed results of this survey will be published at a later date. We also plan to give more information from the many letters that women wrote and sent in with their questionnaires.

Figure 9: Respondents' positive and negative responses to having a hysterectomy

	Responses about feelings at time of hysterectomy		Responses about having had a hysterectomy	
	Positive	Negative	Positive	Negative
1. Health and general condition	33 (3%)	147 (15%)	265 (27%)	49 (5%)
2. Health care system	25 (3%)	107 (11%)	12 (1%)	93 (9%)
3. Support systems	50 (5%)	2	0	3
4. Feelings about the operation	530 (64%)	434 (44%)	840 (85%)	297 (30%)
5. Self image	0	41 (4%)	30 (3%)	32 (3%)
6. Personal relationships and sexuality	0	21 (2%)	26 (3%)	82 (8%)
7. Fertility	0	6	0	36 (4%)

HYSTERECTOMY QUESTIONNAIRE

1. Age _____

2. No of children _____

3. Are you Maori ☐
            Pakeha ☐
            Pacific Islander ☐
            Other ☐

4. What year did you have your hysterectomy? _____

5. What was removed? _____

6. Why did you have a hysterectomy? (Please tick as many boxes as apply.)
   Cancer ☐
   Fibroids ☐
   Endometriosis ☐
   Infection ☐
   Heavy bleeding ☐
   Prolapse/or repair ☐
   Problems after sterilisation ☐
   Problems after contraceptive use,
   e.g. IUD or Depo Provera ☐
   As a method of sterilisation ☐
   Other ☐

7. Did you feel you were given enough information by your doctor to agree to the operation?
   Yes ☐   No ☐

8. Did your doctor inform you of any possible negative effects of the hysterectomy?
   Yes ☐   No ☐

   If yes, which of the following? (Tick as many as apply.)
   Depression ☐
   Mood swings ☐
   Infection ☐
   Haemorrhage ☐
   Bladder or bowel problems ☐
   Difficulty reaching orgasm ☐
   Less satisfactory sex life ☐
   Hot flushes ☐
   Other ☐

9. Did you experience any negative effects as a result of the hysterectomy?
   Yes ☐   No ☐

If yes, which of the following? (Tick as many as apply.)
Depression ☐
Mood swings ☐
Infection ☐
Haemorrhage ☐
Bladder or bowel problems ☐
Difficulty reaching orgasm ☐
Less satisfactory sex life ☐
Hot flushes ☐
Grief at loss of fertility ☐
Feeling incomplete as a woman ☐
Regret at loss of menstruation ☐
Other ☐

10. Did you experience any positive effects of the hysterectomy?
Yes ☐   No ☐

If yes, which of the following? (Tick as many as apply.)
Relief of symptoms ☐
Increased sexual pleasure ☐
Improved physical health ☐
Improved psychological health ☐
Freedom from periods ☐
Other ☐

11. Following your hysterectomy did you receive any further treatment?
Yes ☐   No ☐

If yes, which of the following? (Tick as many as apply.)
Oestrogen replacement therapy ☐
Corrective surgery ☐
Treatment for depression ☐
Sexual counselling ☐
Antibiotics ☐
Other ☐

12. Please describe your feelings at the time of the hysterectomy. (Use extra paper if necessary.)

_____

_____

13. How do you feel now about having had a hysterectomy? (Use extra paper if necessary.)

_____

_____

Thank you for helping.

GLOSSARY

Acute	Sudden.
Adhesion	Surfaces stuck together with scar tissue.
Benign	Harmless.
Biopsy	Sample of tissue.
Cancer precursor	Condition that could lead to cancer if untreated.
Carcinoma in situ	Abnormal cells in cervix, which if untreated can lead to invasive cancer.
Catheter	Tube passed into the bladder to drain it.
Cervix	Neck of the womb protruding into the vagina.
Cervical cancer	Cancer of the cervix that is invading deeper cells.
Cervical intraepithelial neoplasia or CIN	Abnormal cervical cells graded CIN 1, CIN 2 or CIN 3. CIN 3 is the same as carcinoma in situ.
Chemotherapy	Drug treatment for cancer.
Chlamydia	Sexually transmitted bacteria causing PID in women.
Chronic	Persistent, recurrent.
Colposcopy	Examination of the cervix under magnification.
Cone biopsy	Cone-shaped piece cut from cervix to remove abnormal cells.
Cyst	A sac or capsule containing liquid or semi-solid substance. Can grow in many parts of the body. Most cysts are harmless.

Cystitis	Painful infection caused by bacteria in the bladder.
Cystocele	Prolapse of the bladder.
Danazol	Drug given to reduce or stop menstruation. Used particularly with endometriosis.
Diathermy	Removal of damaged or diseased tissue by burning.
Dilatation and curettage (D & C)	Stretching open the canal through the cervix and scraping out the lining of the uterus.
Ectopic pregnancy	Pregnancy in the Fallopian tube.
Endocrinologist	One who studies hormones, and the glands that secrete them.
Endometrial biopsy	Sample taken from endometrium to check for disease.
Endometrial hyperplasia	Overgrowth of endometrium. Can be benign or pre-cancerous.
Endometriosis	Disease where fragments of endometrium grow in places other than inside the uterus. Can lead to cysts, called chocolate cysts.
Endometrium	Lining of uterus, which comes away monthly as a menstrual period.
Epithelium	Tissue covering the body's external surface and lining hollow structures such as the cervix.
Fallopian tubes	Tubes leading from the uterus to the ovaries.
Fibroids	Lumps of fibrous tissue which develop in the normal muscle of the uterus. They are not cancerous.
Fistula	An abnormal hole between two organs.
Haemorrhage	Sudden, excessive bleeding.

Histology	Tissue diagnosis.
Hormone replacement therapy (HRT)	Oestrogen and progesterone given for menopausal symptoms and pre-menstrual tension.
Hot flush	Sudden feeling of heat and sweating experienced by women during menopause.
Hysterectomy	Surgical removal of the uterus.
Intravenous	Into a vein.
Laser	Treatment for various conditions that destroys diseased cells by vaporising them. Causes minimal bleeding and good healing results.
Libido	Interest in sex.
Lymph nodes	Part of the drainage system of the body.
Malignant	Cancerous.
Menopause	Change of life or climacteric. Period of a woman's life marked by the end of menstruation and sometimes other symptoms such as hot flushes. Surgical menopause is caused by removal of the ovaries as oestrogen production is ended.
Myomectomy	Operation to cut out fibroids.
Obese	Very overweight.
Oestrogen	A female sex hormone, produced in the ovaries. It is responsible for female secondary sexual characteristic development, the health of the genital organs and, with progesterone, for menstruation.
Oestrogen replacement therapy (ERT)	Hormones given to increase oestrogen in menopausal women or women suffering from premenstrual tension.

Oophorectomy	Removal of an ovary. Removal of both ovaries is called bilateral oophorectomy.
Osteoporosis	Thinning of the bones leading to fractures.
Ovaries	Small organs on both sides of the pelvis, which produce eggs and manufacture hormones.
Pathology	Diagnosis of disease from tissue.
Pelvic inflammatory disease (PID)	Persistent infection in the pelvic organs.
Pelvis	Basin-like structure of bones containing a woman's reproductive organs.
Peritoneum	Smooth thin material covering the outside of the uterus.
Pre-cancer	A condition which could lead to cancer if untreated.
Progesterone	Hormone produced by the ovaries. Helps produce the lining of the uterus.
Progestin or progestogen	Artificial or synthetic progesterone.
Prolapse	Dropping of body organ.
Pulmonary embolism	Blocking of pulmonary artery, usually by a blood clot.
Pyometra	Build-up of pus in the uterus, often caused by disease.
Radiation therapy	The application of radiation, by X-ray or radioactive substances, to treat cancer.
Rectocele	Abnormal condition where part of rectum bulges into the vagina.
Testosterone	Male hormone also secreted by women.

Thrombosis	Formation of blood clot.
Tumour	Swelling or new abnormal growth of tissue.
Ureter	Tube from kidney to bladder for carrying urine.
Urethra	Tube for carrying urine from bladder to exterior.
Urethrocele	Prolapse of the urethra.
Uterus	Womb. The reproductive organ that carries a child to term and that bleeds monthly until menopause.
Vagina	Canal from uterus to the outside of a woman's body.
Wertheim's hysterectomy	Removal of the uterus, part of the vagina and other pelvic tissue as a treatment for cancer. Also combined with radiation therapy.
Womb	Uterus.

BIBLIOGRAPHY

Books

Dennerstein, Lorraine *et al. Hysterectomy*. Melbourne, 1982.
Dyson, Linda. *Cervical Cancer*. Auckland, 1986.
Haines, Hilary. *Mental Health For Women*. Auckland, 1987.
Hayman, Suzie. *Hysterectomy*. London, 1986.
Hufnagel, Vicki. *No More Hysterectomies*. New York, 1988.
Kahn, Ada and Holt, Linda. *Menopause: The Best Years of Your Life?* London, 1987.
Keyser, Herbert H. *Women Under the Knife*. Philadelphia, 1984.
Madaras, Lynda and Patterson, Jane. *Womancare*. New York, 1984.
McKenzie, Raewyn. *Menopause*. Auckland, 1984.
Morgan, Susanne. *Hysterectomy*. Washington, 1980.
Reitz, Rosetta. *Menopause: A Positive Approach*. London, 1985.

Books on sexuality

Boston Women's Health Book Collective. *The New Our Bodies, Ourselves*. New York, 1987.
Cartledge, S. and Ryan, J. eds. *Sex and Love: New Thoughts on Old Contradictions*. London, 1983.
Dickson, A. *The Mirror Within: A New Look at Sexuality*. London, 1985.
Eichenbaum, L. and Orbach, S. *What Do Women Want?* London, 1982.
Gray, A. *Expressions of Sexuality*. Auckland, 1985.
Hepburn, G. and Gutirrez, B. *Alive and Well: A Lesbian Health Guide*. Freedom, California, 1988.

Hite, S. *Women and Love*. London, 1988.

Kerr, C. *Sex for Women*. New York, 1978.

Kitzinger, S. *Women's Experience of Sex*. Sydney, 1984.

Loulan, J. *Lesbian Passion: Loving Ourselves and Each Other*. San Francisco, 1987.

Woods, M. F. *Human Sexuality in Health and Illness*. St Louis, 1979.

Articles and papers (selection)

Barter, Robert H. *et al*. 'Vaginal versus Abdominal Hysterectomy.' In Reid, D. and Christian II, C. D., eds, *Controversy in Obstetrics and Gynaecology*, Philadelphia, 1974.

Bell, J. *et al*. 'Vaginal cancer after hysterectomy for benign disease: value of cytologic screening.' *Obstetrics and Gynaecology*, November 1984: 699–702.

Bernhard, Linda Ann. 'Black Women's Concerns about Sexuality and Hysterectomy.' *SAGE*, Vol. II No. 2, Fall 1985: 25–27.

Borman, Barry *et al*. 'Hysterectomies in New Zealand.' Letter to *New Zealand Medical Journal*, 25 June 1986: 470.

Cattanach, J. 'Oestrogen Deficiency after Tubal Ligation.' *The Lancet*, 13 April 1985: 847–849.

Cohen, Marsha M. 'Long-term Risks of Hysterectomy after Tubal Ligation.' *American Journal of Epidemiology*, Vol. 125 No. 3, 1987: 410–19.

Colditz, Graham A. *et al*. 'Menopause and the Risk of Coronary Heart Disease in Women.' *New England Journal of Medicine*, Vol. 316 No. 18, 30 April 1987: 1105–1110.

Coulter, Angela *et al*. 'Do British Women Undergo Too Many or Too Few Hysterectomies?' *Social Science and Medicine*, Vol. 27 No. 9, 1988: 987–94.

Dennerstein, L. and Ryan, M. 'Psycho-Social and Emotional Sequelae of Hysterectomy.' *Journal of Psycho-Somatic Obstetrics and Gynaecology*, Vol. 1 - 2, 1982: 81–86.

Domenighetti, G. *et al.* 'Hysterectomy and Sex of the Gynaecologist.' Letter to the *New England Journal of Medicine*, 5 December 1985: 1482.

Gath, D. *et al.* 'Hysterectomy and Psychiatric Disorder: I.' *International Journal of Psychiatry*, Vol. 140, 1982: 335.

Gould, Dinah. 'Understanding Emotional Need.' *Nursing Mirror*, Vol. 160, 2 January 1985: 2–8.

Greenwood, Sadja. 'Update on Hysterectomy, Ovarian Removal and Androgen Replacement.' *PMZ Newsletter*, Fall 1985.

Helms, Joseph M. 'Acupuncture for the Management of Primary Dysmenorrhoea.' *Obstetrics and Gynaecology*, Vol. 69 No. 1, January 1987: 51–56.

Jackson, Peter. 'Sexual Adjustment to Hysterectomy and the Benefits of a Pamphlet for Patients.' *New Zealand Medical Journal*, 12 December 1979: 471–72.

Loffer, Franklin D. 'Hysteroscopic Endometrial Ablation with the ND: YAG Laser Using a Nontouch Technique.' *Obstetrics and Gynaecology*, Vol. 69 No. 4, April 1987: 679–82.

MacDonald, Paul C. 'Estrogen Plus Progestine in Postmenopausal Women — Act II.' *New England Journal of Medicine*, Vol. 315 No. 15, 9 October 1986: 959–61.

Macintosh, Mary C. 'Incidence of Hysterectomy in New Zealand.' *New Zealand Medical Journal*, 10 June 1987: 345–47.

McKinlay, John B. *et al.* 'The Relative Contributions of Endocrine Changes and Social Circumstances to Depression in Mid-Aged Women.' New England Research Institute, Massachusetts, research paper, undated.

Morgan, Susanne. 'Sex after Hysterectomy: What Your Doctor Never Told You.' *Ms Magazine*, March 1982: 82–85.

Napoli, Maryann. 'Medical Breakthrough: Laser Hysterectomy.' *Ms Magazine*, March 1986: 30–33.

New York State Department of Health. 'Hysterectomies in New York State: A Statistical Profile.' June 1988: 13.

Ngu, A. and Quinn M. A. 'Dysfunctional Uterine Bleeding in Women over 40 Years of Age.' *Australia New Zealand Journal of Obstetrics and Gynaecology*, 1984, Vol. 24 No. 30: 30–33.

Opit, L. J. and Gadiel, David. 'Hysterectomy in New South Wales: An Evaluation of Its Use and Outcome.' Office of Health Care Finance. Sydney, 1982.

Punnonen, R. *et al.* 'Premenopausal Hysterectomy and Risk of Cardiovascular Disease.' *The Lancet*, 16 May 1987: 1139.

Richards, D. H. 'Depression after Hysterectomy.' *The Lancet*, 25 October 1973: 430–32.

Richards, D. H. 'A Post-Hysterectomy Syndrome.' *The Lancet*, 26 October 1974: 983–85.

Riedel, H. *et al.* 'Ovarian Failure after Hysterectomy.' *The Journal of Reproductive Medicine*, Vol. 31 No. 7, July 1986: 597–600.

Roos, Noralou P. 'Hysterectomies in One Canadian Province: A New Look at Risks and Benefits.' *American Journal of Public Health*, Vol. 74 No. 1, January 1984: 39–45.

Roos, Noralou P. 'Hysterectomy: Variations in Rates across Small Areas and across Physicians' Practices.' *American Journal of Public Health*, Vol. 74 No. 4, April 1984: 327–34.

Ryan, Margaret. 'Psychosexual Aspects of Hysterectomy.' Ph.D. thesis, University of Melbourne, 1985.

Shapiro, Mervyn *et al.* 'Risk Factors for Infection at the Operative Site after Abdominal or Vaginal Hysterectomy.' *New England Journal of Medicine*, Vol. 307 No. 27, 30 December 1982: 1661–66.

Sloan, Don. 'The Emotional and Psychosexual Aspects of Hysterectomy.' *American Journal of Obstetrics and Gynaecology*, Vol. 131 No. 6, 15 July 1987: 598–605.

US Department of Health and Human Services. *Hysterectomy in the United States, 1965–1984*. December 1987.

Wilkinson, E. J. and Mattingly, R. F. 'Medical versus Surgical

Management of Endometriosis.' In Reid, D. and Christian II, C.D. eds, *Controversy in Obstetrics and Gynaecology*, Philadelphia, 1974.

Wren, B. G. 'Oestrogen Therapy after Menopause: A Viewpoint on its Rational Use.' *Current Therapeutics*, March 1987: 25–36.

Zussman, Leon *et al.* 'Sexual Response after Hysterectomy-oophorectomy: Recent Studies and Reconsideration of Psychogenesis.' *American Journal of Obstetrics and Gynaecology*, Vol. 140 No. 7, 1 August 1981: 725–730.

INDEX